Disclaimer

Summary

Introduction:

Is it finally time to say, "Enough is enough"? Are you ready to embark on a journey to a healthier version of yourself, with no more excuses, making a real change and losing those extra pounds... No matter what!

If you find yourself in this situation, be prepared to...

Hug the **fat-act** and radically transform your life!

Saturday morning and late night infomercials . They promote gadgets and gimmicks that promise quick and easy weight loss. How many of us have seen those "magic abs" that we sit on and rock on while the fat seems to melt away like snow in the sun? The reality, unfortunately, is quite different.

Have you ever read the fine print at the bottom of the screen during these ads? Well, it basically tells you that you have to follow some form of strict diet for these miracle products to be even slightly effective. It's a crucial detail that often gets overlooked.

In today's digital age, it's all too easy to fall for the alluring promises of rapid weight loss offered by fancy diet plans, "magic diet pills," or other so-called "miracle weight loss diets." But honestly, there are some basic truths you should know before making a decision that could profoundly impact your health and well -being.

First of all, you need to realize that there is NO miracle weight loss treatment. While it is possible to lose significant weight by adhering to highly restrictive or popular fad diets, the truth is that they are not sustainable in the long term and can even be harmful to your health.

In addition to the obvious negative side effects on your physical and mental health, I have found that the word "diet" immediately conjures up a sense of restriction and deprivation in my mind. If you look at the dictionary, one of the definitions of "diet" is: "a restrictive eating regimen designed to reduce weight." It is no surprise then that traditional diets often fail in the long run!

The latest scientific studies unequivocally demonstrate that most overweight people who embark on crash diets regain the weight they lost almost immediately, entering a frustrating cycle of weight loss and regain known as the "yo-yo effect." What is even more worrying is that these people are often in worse health than those who maintain their original overweight weight, due to the physical and psychological stress caused by these fluctuations.

If we are honest with each other, the fundamental principles of weight loss have not changed since we began walking this earth. What has changed dramatically is the marketing and merchandising of weight loss strategies. Ultimately , the secret lies in creating a sustainable negative energy balance over time.

But how do you achieve a negative energy balance in a healthy and lasting way? There are three main approaches:

- You can reduce the amount of calories you consume each day by focusing on nutritious, filling foods.
- You can increase the intensity and frequency of your workout sessions, burning more calories through physical activity.
- Ideally, you can combine both approaches, creating a balanced and sustainable calorie deficit.

It's all here, in its simplicity and effectiveness.

That being said... there are no miracles or shortcuts, just scientifically proven nutritional advice and proven exercises, and that is exactly what this book will cover in depth.

The main goal of "Revolutionize Your Body: Burn Fat with Kettlebells" is to eliminate all the falsehoods and myths that circulate on the Internet about weight loss and finally help you make lasting changes to your lifestyle. We will guide you step by step towards achieving the weight goal that you have decided is best for you, providing you with the tools and knowledge necessary to maintain the results in the long term.

This book will teach you how to use kettlebells, a versatile and effective tool, to burn fat and build lean muscle. We will combine functional strength exercises with high- intensity cardio movements, creating a complete workout program that will accelerate your metabolism and transform your body.

Additionally, we will explore sustainable nutritional strategies that fit your lifestyle, without extreme restrictions or deprivation. You'll learn how to make smart food choices that support your fitness goals and improve your overall health.

Today is the day to make the decision to **SAY GOODBYE TO FAT AND CHANGE YOUR LIFE... FOREVER.**

Are you ready to embark on this journey to a stronger, healthier, happier version of yourself? Turn the page and let's start this transformation together!

Chapter 1: "Why am I gaining weight?

In the modern era, characterized by frenetic rhythms, technological advances and the widespread availability of fast food, maintaining an active lifestyle and a balanced diet has become an increasingly complex challenge. However, even in this context , there are effective strategies to preserve one's health and physical fitness.

In the first section of this book, we will delve into the following topics, providing up-to-date information:

- The main factors that contribute to weight gain.
- The professionals to consult when you decide to undertake a weight loss path .
- How to structure and follow an effective weight loss program.
- Advanced techniques and innovative strategies for lasting weight loss.
- more about losing weight permanently and maintaining results long-term.

The causes of weight gain are many and interconnected. The basic principle remains the imbalance between calories consumed and calories burned: when we consume more energy than our body uses, the excess is stored as fat. But why, according to the most recent statistics, are over 65% of Americans overweight or obese? One of the main reasons is the exponential increase in portion sizes in recent decades.

When we eat more food than our body can metabolize, a positive energy balance is created, resulting in the accumulation of fat. This mechanism, advantageous for our ancestors in times of food scarcity, is counterproductive in contemporary Western society, characterized by a constant abundance of food.

weight loss process . Recent studies published in the Canadian Medical Association Journal have highlighted a significant correlation between sleep quality and weight control. It was found that people with irregular sleep habits or who sleep little tend to consume 400 to 500 more calories per day, compromising diet and exercise efforts.

As we age, our metabolism naturally slows down. On average, every decade after the age of 25 , our metabolic rate decreases by about 10%. However, this decline can be effectively counteracted by following the kettlebell training program described in this book. Increasing muscle mass stimulates our metabolism, as the body requires more energy to maintain and repair muscle tissue after exercise. On the other hand, a sedentary lifestyle accelerates the process of weight gain.

Modern eating habits are another critical factor. The latest research indicates that, on average, individuals in Western societies weigh about 33 pounds more than they did a century ago, even though fat consumption has not increased proportionately. The real culprit appears to be the increase in consumption of ultra-processed foods. As fitness pioneer Jack LaLanne wisely put it, "If it's man-made, don't eat it."

Refined sugars, starches, and refined flour products are contributing significantly to the obesity epidemic in our society. In 2023, according to the latest statistics from FastFoodFacts.com, the fast food industry spent over $5 billion on advertising. It is no surprise, then, that there is a high incidence of overweight. Many people have found benefit from using meal planning apps to guide them toward healthier food choices.

Portion sizes have seen significant inflation in recent years. This is especially true in fast food chains, where drinks and side dishes have grown exponentially. Most people, unknowingly, consume far more food than they need. Using meal planning tools can help you understand and stick to proper portion sizes.

Physical activity, or lack thereof, plays a crucial role in the health of Western society. According to projections by DesignedToMove.org, today's children could be the first generation with a life expectancy lower than that of their parents, mainly due to sedentary lifestyles. The human body is designed for movement, and regular exercise is essential not only to achieving and maintaining a healthy weight, but also to overall health. I invite you to follow the innovative program proposed by Sergente Sottile, a fitness expert who is revolutionizing the approach to training to become the fittest man in the world.

Learning to control portion sizes is essential. A practical and effective method, which does not require scales or measuring devices, is to use your hand as a reference. For men, it is recommended to consume 2 servings of protein per meal, while for women 1 serving is sufficient. A serving is approximately the size of the palm of your hand.

For complex carbohydrates, both men and women should stick to a portion about the size of their closed fist. For healthy fats, such as nuts or seeds, the ideal portion is about the size of your thumb.

It is essential to learn to recognize your body's satiety signals. An effective technique is to stop eating when you feel 80% full . By applying this strategy consistently, you can achieve a significant reduction in calorie intake over time, without feeling deprived.

Slowing down during meals is another habit to cultivate. Avoid eating in the car, standing up, or while walking. Focus on your food and eat only at the table. Eating slowly allows your brain to correctly receive satiety signals, reducing the risk of overeating. If your routine is particularly hectic, consider using healthy and balanced meal replacements to maintain a balanced diet even in the busiest moments.

An often overlooked aspect is the impact of high-fat, high-sugar foods. While our bodies require a certain amount of healthy fats to function properly, overconsumption of ultra-processed foods and sugary drinks is directly linked to weight gain. Processed foods tend to be low in nutritional value and high in salt, added sugars, and unhealthy fats.

Many people tend to use their hectic lifestyle as an excuse for gaining weight. In fact, it is precisely in these situations that it becomes crucial to plan ahead to avoid the traps that lead to bad food choices. As a famous bodybuilder said, "Tupperware is a fundamental tool during athletic preparation." This statement is more relevant than ever.

Using a personalized meal planner, like the one available through the link provided, you can organize your weekly meals and receive a detailed grocery list with all the necessary ingredients. Dedicating a few hours on Sunday to preparing meals for the entire week, freezing portions and taking them with you every day, will allow you to eliminate the daily stress related to food choices.

Breakfast, often overlooked or consumed in a hurry, deserves special attention. Instead of opting for unhealthy choices or skipping the meal altogether, consider using balanced meal replacements to start your day off right, staying on track with your health and fitness goals.

Remember that sustainable weight loss is not just about diet, but requires a holistic approach that includes regular exercise, stress management, and adequate sleep. By gradually implementing these strategies into your daily routine, you can overcome the challenges of modern lifestyle and reach your health and wellness goals .

"Do you have to follow a diet?

The short answer is absolutely not. Traditional diets rarely work in the long run. As we've discussed, with the aggressive marketing of the latest "fad diets," it's easy to get caught up in the hype.

This is exactly what Corey Lewis talks about in his book "Sergeant Slim's Mass Reduction Weapons", emphasizing the importance of a sustainable approach to wellness. Instead of thinking about a temporary diet, consider an overall lifestyle change, which will allow you to develop healthy eating and exercise habits in the long term .

It is neither necessary nor advisable to eliminate entire food groups, such as carbohydrates, nor to rely on weight-loss shakes that are neither satisfying nor tasty. Often, people start a diet around specific events, such as a wedding, graduation, or family reunion, or at the start of a new year. If this is your sole goal, I strongly encourage you to do your own research and avoid drastic solutions that will not yield lasting results. Instead, focus on gradual, sustainable changes that you can maintain over time.

In conclusion, don't let a hectic lifestyle get in the way of your desire to lose weight and stay healthy. Plan ahead, pay attention to portion sizes, eat slowly, and make conscious food choices. Be consistent with your exercise, including kettlebell workouts as suggested in the book, and make sure you get the quality sleep you need. Remember, lifestyle changes take time and patience, but the results will be long-lasting and incredibly rewarding. Good luck on your journey to a healthier, more active life!

Set goals... Think SMART

Before we undertake any kind of change in our normal daily life, it is essential to have a clear and compelling reason why we are doing it. These are our goals, and their importance cannot be underestimated.

Goals are crucial because they give us the motivation we need when the going gets tough. Maybe you recently went from a size 10 to a size 12 and are tired of feeling weighed down. Or maybe your doctor has warned you that you need to lose 20 pounds to avoid serious health problems. Whatever your situation, it is essential that your goals are real and meaningful to you.

To make your goals tangible and accessible, I recommend writing them down and placing them somewhere you can see them every day. This simple act of daily visualization can have a powerful impact on your motivation and determination. My favorite formula to use for setting effective goals is the SMART acronym:

Specific : If you only have a vague idea of your goal, you're likely to fail before you even start. Think about it: If you were driving to New York City, you wouldn't get in the car without specific directions, right ? Likewise, a generic statement like

"I want to get in shape" isn't specific enough. It has no concrete meaning, and you won't even know if you've reached your goal. Why? Because even if you only lost a pound, you'd technically be in better shape than where you started.

It's important to be specific and define exactly what you want to achieve. For example, a goal like "I want to lose 30 pounds and be able to wear my college pants by the end of the year" is much clearer and more measurable. Notice the difference? With this type of specific goal, you'll have a clear end point and can track your progress along the way.

Measurable : This aspect is closely related to the specificity of the goal. Your goal must be quantifiable in some way. What does this mean ? Make sure your statement answers questions like "how much?" or "how many?" In the example above, the answer would be "15 kilos".

It's also helpful to set milestones along the way to track your progress. For example, you might say, "I want to lose 30 pounds in total, which means I need to lose about 2.5 pounds every month for a year." This approach will help you track your progress and stay motivated. As the old Chinese proverb says, "A journey of a thousand miles begins with a single step." You can't lose 30 pounds all at once, but you can certainly lose a pound this week!

Attainable : This criterion is fairly intuitive, but it is crucial to keep your goal within the realm of reason. Don't expect to hop on the treadmill once and lose ten pounds in a day! Instead, you need to break your goal down into smaller milestones that are ambitious enough to make you work hard, but also achievable.

If you set goals that are too ambitious , after a few weeks of not meeting your expectations, you may become discouraged and give up altogether. It would be better to set your initial goal more moderately and then gradually increase it as you consistently exceed your weekly milestones. This approach will allow you to build confidence and momentum in your transformation journey.

Realistic : An attainable goal is inherently realistic , but there is a subtle difference between the two. It may be theoretically possible to reach a certain goal, but you may not be willing or able to do so in your current life circumstances. For example, while reducing body fat to 7 percent may be physically possible in theory, it may not be realistic for most people, given their lifestyle, genetics, and other factors.

40 pounds overweight , your initial goal should be to get into a reasonable and sustainable shape. Trying to go from your current condition to the fitness level of a professional athlete is not truly realistic and could lead to frustration down the road.

Just because a goal is possible (attainable) doesn't necessarily mean you have a reasonable chance of success (realistic) in your current context . So , try to keep your goal somewhere in the middle and you'll have a better chance of success! A good statement might be: "I want to reduce my body fat percentage from 22 to 16 percent in seven months by incorporating regular kettlebell workouts and improving my nutrition."

However, remember that a challenging goal can make your task easier, because it will keep you motivated. Setting the bar too low can make you feel unmotivated. Only you can decide where the right balance is for you, and you can always raise the bar halfway if you feel like you need more of a challenge!

Time-bound : You've probably noticed that each example includes a specific time frame . This is essential, otherwise you won't know how to plan along the way and may procrastinate indefinitely. If you give yourself 2 years to lose 20 pounds, then you should aim to lose less than a pound per month. However, if you plan to achieve the same goal in just one year, you'll need to double that pace.

Your deadline is therefore a key part of your goal and should be very specific. Make sure you choose a timeframe that is both challenging and realistic, considering your lifestyle and commitments. Remember that you can always adjust your timeframe along the way if you find that your initial pace was too ambitious or too cautious.

Relevant : Last but not least, the goal must be relevant and meaningful to you on a personal level. It must have intrinsic value and a tangible impact on your life. Before committing to a goal, honestly ask yourself why you want to achieve it and what tangible benefits you will get once you have achieved it.

and emotional connection to your goal is essential to keep you motivated throughout the process, especially when you encounter obstacles or difficult moments. A goal that is truly relevant to you will push you to overcome challenges and persevere even when the going gets tough.

Remember, the journey to a healthier, fitter life is not just about the numbers on the scale or your body measurements. It's about improving your overall quality of life, increasing your energy, strengthening your health, and feeling more confident and satisfied with yourself. By using the SMART method of setting your goals, combined with the innovative approach to kettlebell training presented in the book "Revolutionize Your Body: Burn Fat with Kettlebells," you'll be on your way to a lasting and meaningful transformation."

Now what?

Now that you have a specific and challenging goal , and you have invested time and energy into making it truly engaging, what is the next step and how can you best leverage it to maximize your results? As already mentioned , it is crucial to reinforce this goal daily, keeping it visible in a strategic location where you will frequently cross your gaze. This practice will constantly remind you of what you are trying to achieve and can be a powerful catalyst for developing new healthy habits.

Behavioral change science suggests that it takes about 66 days to solidify a new habit, not just the 21 days previously mentioned. So , after about two months of consistent commitment to balanced nutrition and regular physical activity, you will notice that your new lifestyle will become more natural and automatic. This will make the journey to your goals much smoother and more sustainable in the long run.

However, if you've been struggling with your weight for years or even decades, you may find yourself deeply entrenched in a sedentary lifestyle and unhealthy eating patterns that seem nearly impossible to break. In these cases, you may need to take a more aggressive and innovative approach to break these harmful cycles and establish new, positive patterns!

An effective strategy might be to accompany your written goal with concrete documents that highlight the consequences of maintaining the status quo. These might include recent medical reports, blood test results that show abnormal values, or a detailed memo from your doctor about your current health status. While this may seem like a brutal approach, if your health is the primary motivation for finally losing weight, it is essential to confront reality directly and honestly.

Viewing this objective data daily can provide unprecedented motivation. You will be constantly reminded of the vital importance of your commitment and the non-negotiability of your health goal. This "shock" approach can be especially effective for those who tend to procrastinate or minimize the urgency of change.

On the other hand, if your motivation is more aesthetic or social, you might opt for a more positive, aspirational visual approach. For example, if your goal is to wear a smaller size to an upcoming event, why not display a photo of the desired item of clothing, or even the dress itself, in a prominent spot in your home?

This visualization technique, based on the principles of positive psychology and "vision boarding ," may seem simplistic, but it is supported by numerous studies on the effectiveness of guided imagery in achieving goals. Having a tangible and visual representation of your goal can make it much easier to resist the daily temptations you may encounter at work, during social outings, or in times of stress.

When you're tempted to deviate from your balanced diet or skip your workout routine, the image of that dress or healthier version of yourself will be fresh in your mind, providing an immediate emotional reminder of why you've embarked on this journey. This simple but powerful psychological tool can make the difference between giving in to a momentary temptation and sticking to your guns.

Get Support: Building an Effective Support Network

At this point in your journey, you may feel like you've done everything you need to ensure your success by defining a SMART (Specific, Measurable, Achievable, Realistic, Time-bound) goal and strategically placing it in a visible location. While these are fundamental and commendable steps, there's one more crucial element you need to consider to maximize your chances of long-term success!

Many people, despite the best of intentions and solid planning up front, fail to achieve their health and fitness goals because they underestimate the importance of a strong support system. This support network becomes essential in the truly difficult moments, when motivation falters and the temptation to abandon the weight loss journey becomes almost irresistible.

It is essential to identify and actively involve people who not only care about you, but who fully understand and support your efforts to improve your health and well-being. Ideally, your partner or spouse would be a key figure in this support system, since you share the day-to-day and, likely, most of the meals. Their involvement can create a cohesive home environment that is conducive to change.

However, the reality is often more complex . Unfortunately, it is not uncommon for your partner to be unwilling to change their habits or, worse, to unknowingly or actively hinder your weight loss plan. This can happen for a variety of reasons: maybe they are also overweight and do not feel ready to face a change, or they simply do not fully understand the importance of this goal for you.

In these cases, it becomes even more crucial to seek strong and constant support outside of the home environment. Close friends, family members or colleagues who share your values of health and well-being can become valuable allies, compensating for the lack of support at home and providing that extra push you need in times of difficulty.

One particularly effective strategy is to seek the help and guidance of a friend or acquaintance who is already in good physical shape and maintaining a healthy lifestyle. This person not only understands the challenges and rewards of maintaining a healthy weight, but can also serve as an inspiring role model and source of practical advice based on firsthand experience.

Additionally, working with someone who has already established healthy habits reduces the risk of negative influences. They won't be tempted to skip workouts or indulge in unhealthy meals, providing a constant example of discipline and consistency. They can also help you stay accountable by gently reminding you of your goals when you might be tempted to give in.

If you don't know anyone who fits this profile in your immediate social circle, consider finding a "fitness buddy" to share this transformation journey with. This partnership can be incredibly motivating : knowing you have a regular date with someone at the gym or for an outdoor workout makes it much harder to find excuses to skip exercise.

Additionally, the mutual accountability that develops in these partnerships can extend beyond physical training. Sharing diet progress, swapping healthy recipes, and openly discussing challenges can create a powerful emotional and practical support system. Knowing that you will be "accountable" to someone else for your food choices can provide that extra incentive to stick to your nutrition plan, even in the face of temptation.

Get a Free Personal Trainer: Take Advantage of Available Resources

In addition to building a strong personal support network, you can further amplify your wellness journey by taking advantage of accessible professional resources. In this context , my experience as a certified personal trainer can represent a valuable and free resource at your disposal.

Through this book and the additional resources I offer online, you have access to a wealth of expert knowledge about nutrition, kettlebell training, and effective weight loss strategies. Feel free to use this information to customize your approach and maximize your results.

Additionally, consider using fitness and nutrition tracking apps, many of which offer free features that can act as a "virtual personal trainer." These apps can help you track your progress, provide workout reminders, and offer personalized nutrition advice.

Put it all together: Summarize your winning strategy

Now that you have all the key elements at your disposal, it's time to synthesize them into a cohesive and powerful strategy. You've learned how to set a solid and motivating goal , following the SMART criteria to ensure that it is specific, measurable, attainable, realistic and time-bound.

Remember to review and reinforce this goal daily, keeping it visually present in your life. Whether it's a reminder of your health or an aspirational image, this visual anchor will be a powerful ally on your journey.

You've learned the critical importance of surrounding yourself with a strong, positive support system . Whether it's your partner, a fit friend, or a fitness buddy, make sure you have someone who can support you, motivate you, and keep you accountable.

Finally, remember to take advantage of all the resources available to you, including the professional knowledge offered in this book and modern technologies that can facilitate your path.

With all of these factors aligned, you will have a clear vision of your destination and the steps needed to get there. Stay consistent, celebrate the small successes along the way, and remember that every day is an opportunity to get closer to your goal of a healthier, fitter body through effective kettlebell use and a balanced lifestyle.

The journey to a better version of yourself starts now. Are you ready to revolutionize your body and your life? "

How Diets Work: A Complete Guide to Sustainable Weight Loss

Losing weight is a fundamentally simple process: you have to consume fewer calories than your body requires on a daily basis. However, the simplicity of this concept does not always translate into ease of execution. Let's see together how to make this path more effective and sustainable.

Balance : The Key to Understanding Body Weight

Eating a balanced diet is essential to keeping our bodies healthy and functioning. However, when we consume more food than we need, we inevitably gain weight. Consider this scenario: if we eat just 300 extra calories a day, over the course of a year we could gain over 20 kilos of weight! This phenomenon is known as positive energy balance: we consume more calories than our body actually needs.

Recent research in nutrition has shown that not all calories are created equal. The types of foods we consume can affect our metabolism, hormone levels, and even the composition of our gut microbiome. These factors, in turn , can affect our ability to burn fat and maintain a healthy weight.

The role of a balanced diet

An effective diet should help you cut excess calories, but not only that. It should also provide all the essential nutrients your body needs. Think of a diet as an eating plan where you carefully control not only the amount of calories you consume, but also the quality of the nutrients you consume.

It is important to dispel the myth that you can eat unlimited amounts of fruits and vegetables just because they are healthy foods. Although these foods are rich in essential nutrients, they still contain calories. The key is to balance your overall caloric intake with the nutrient density of the foods you choose.

In 2024, the use of apps and wearables for tracking nutrition and physical activity has become increasingly sophisticated. These tools can help you track not only calories, but also nutritional composition of your meals, giving you a more complete view of your diet.

Strategies for managing hunger

Many people fear that they will feel unbearably hungry when they drastically reduce their calorie intake. This can happen, but there are effective strategies to manage this feeling. Eating frequent meals, every 2-4 hours, can help minimize the feeling of hunger. A practical approach is to divide the number of hours you are awake by three. For example, if you are awake for 15 hours a day, your goal should be to eat 5 meals.

The latest research in chronobiology has shown that meal timing can be just as important as calorie content. Consuming the majority of calories early in the day, when our metabolism is most active, can lead to better results in terms of weight loss and metabolic health.

Additionally, including high-fiber and high-protein foods in each meal can increase satiety and reduce overall hunger. Protein, in particular, has been shown to have a higher thermogenic effect than carbohydrates and fats, meaning the body burns more calories when digesting protein.

Managing Unforeseen Situations

In everyday life, there may be situations where it is not possible to eat a regular meal. In these cases, a meal replacement can be an effective solution to stay on track with your meal plan. In 2024, increasingly sophisticated meal replacement options are available, which not only provide an adequate caloric intake, but also a complete nutritional profile, including essential micronutrients and fiber.

It is important to avoid skipping meals, especially in the initial phase of the diet plan. This can lead to a phenomenon that experts call "compensation," in which you psychologically tend to overeat at the next meal, undermining your calorie control efforts.

Long-term sustainability

The main reason why many people fail with diets is that they are often too restrictive or unsustainable in the long term. It is unrealistic to think that you can drink only water and eat only vegetables for extended periods of time. A more effective approach is to create a personalized meal plan that takes into account your food preferences, lifestyle, and health goals.

The latest research has shown that dietary flexibility is crucial to long-term success. This approach, known as "flexible eating" or "IIFYM" (If It Fits Your Macros), allows you to include a variety of foods, including those traditionally considered "non-diet," as long as they fit into your overall calorie and nutritional plan.

The Importance of Meal Planning

A personalized meal planner is a critical tool for diet success. It takes the guesswork out of what to eat to lose weight and provides a clear structure to follow. With the advent of AI and machine learning, meal planners in 2024 can dynamically adapt to your preferences, progress, and even health status, offering increasingly personalized suggestions.

Discipline and consistency

Discipline remains one of the most critical factors when trying to stick to a long-term diet plan. Losing weight through proper nutrition takes months or even years to achieve and maintain your desired weight. Crash diets that promise quick results often lead to the yo-yo effect, where you lose weight quickly but gain it back just as quickly, often in greater quantities.

To avoid this, it is essential to adopt a holistic approach to health, which includes not only a balanced diet, but also regular exercise, stress management and adequate sleep. The most recent research has highlighted how these factors are interconnected and can influence each other in determining the success of a weight loss program.

The role of social support

Changing your eating habits often requires the support of your partner or significant others in your life. Studies have shown that social support can significantly increase your chances of success in a weight loss program. Involving those close to you in your new eating plan can create a more supportive environment for change and can also bring health benefits to those around you.

In 2024, social media platforms and fitness apps offer new opportunities to connect with communities of like-minded people, providing support, motivation, and accountability to one another.

Variety and flexibility

An effective meal planner should offer a wide variety of food combinations. Monotony in dieting is one of the main factors that lead to abandonment of weight loss programs. Having a variety of foods available, including those you enjoy, will increase your chances of sticking to the plan in the long run.

The latest trends in personalized nutrition are exploring how genetic differences and the gut microbiome can influence individual responses to different foods. This could lead to even more personalized and effective dietary recommendations in the future.

Error Management and Resilience

It's important to remember that perfection isn't necessary for success . If you occasionally slip up and have a meal or two that throws off your calorie count for the day, the important thing is to get back on track the next day. The goal is to be consistent 90% of the time. A small weekly cheat won't significantly compromise your weight loss goals.

Research on the psychology of behavior change has shown that resilience and the ability to bounce back from mistakes are crucial to long-term success. Developing strategies to manage setbacks and maintaining a positive mindset is just as important as sticking to the meal plan itself.

Industry Secrets

In the world of weight loss and fitness, there are many hidden truths that the industry prefers not to reveal. Their prosperity is often based on fads, catchy gadgets, and miracle solutions sold to people who want to lose weight quickly. Unfortunately, most of these methods prove ineffective, with only a small percentage of buyers actually achieving and maintaining their weight goals.

Here are some industry secrets you should know:

1. Deception in weight loss product ads

Most weight loss products advertised in the media promise unrealistic results. Phrases like "Lose weight effortlessly," " Eat what you want and lose weight," or "No diet or exercise required" are common but deceptive. Always remember: if it seems too good to be true, it probably is.

2. The Deception of "Scientificly Proven" Claims

Many products claim to be "scientifically proven" or "doctor approved." However, details about the studies conducted or the experts involved are often missing. In many cases, the "experts" cited have a financial interest in the product, compromising the objectivity of their assessments. Don't put your health at risk by blindly trusting these claims.

3. Government approval is no guarantee of effectiveness

Contrary to popular belief, government approval of a product does not automatically guarantee its safety or effectiveness. Many "natural" or "herbal" products are allowed to be marketed freely until the FDA receives concrete evidence that they are dangerous. Always use caution and do thorough research before using any new product.

4. The myth of fad diets

Diets that promise drastic changes in a short time are difficult to maintain and often counterproductive. The cycle of rapid weight loss followed by rapid recovery can make it more difficult to lose weight in the future. Instead, look for balanced and sustainable long-term approaches.

5. The Illusion of Money Back Guarantees

Many companies offer seemingly enticing money-back guarantees, but in practice, getting a refund can be difficult. Be wary of products that promise miraculous results with money-back guarantees that are too good to be true.

6. The Power of Kettlebell Training

best- kept secrets in the fitness world is the extraordinary effectiveness of kettlebell training for weight loss. These versatile tools offer a complete workout that combines cardio and strength, boosting your metabolism and burning fat more efficiently than traditional exercises.

7. Benefits of Kettlebells for Weight Loss:

- **Calorie Burn** : An intense kettlebell workout can burn up to 20 calories per minute.
- **Elevated EPOC** : Excess Post-exercise Oxygen Consumption remains high for hours after your workout, continuing to burn calories.
- **Functional Training** : Improves strength, stability and mobility in everyday movements.
- **Time saving** : Short but intense training sessions for fast results.

8. The Importance of Nutrition in Kettlebell Training

To maximize the results of your kettlebell workout, it is essential to combine it with proper nutrition. A balanced, protein-rich meal plan supports muscle growth and fat loss.

- **Nutritional Strategies to Optimize Kettlebell Training:**
- **Meal Timing** : Consume protein and complex carbohydrates before and after your workout.

- **Hydration** : Drink enough water to support your metabolism and performance.
- **Anti-Inflammatory Foods** : Include foods rich in omega-3s and antioxidants to aid recovery.

9. The Winning Mindset for Body Transformation

Weight loss and fitness success depends not only on physical training, but also on mental strength. Developing a resilient mindset is crucial to overcoming obstacles and staying motivated in the long run.

Techniques to develop a winning mindset:

- **Visualization** : Vividly imagine your ideal body and your achieved goals.
- **Positive Affirmations** : Repeat motivational mantras during your workout.
- **Progress Tracking** : Celebrate every small milestone to keep yourself motivated.

10. The importance of recovery and sleep

Often overlooked, proper recovery is key to optimizing kettlebell training and weight loss results. Quality sleep is essential for hormone regulation and muscle recovery.

Strategies for optimal recovery:

- **Regular Sleep** : Aim for 7-9 hours of quality sleep every night.
- **Relaxation techniques** : Practice meditation or yoga to reduce stress.
- **Post-Workout Nutrition** : Consume protein and carbohydrates within 30 minutes of training to aid recovery.

11. Smart integration into kettlebell training

While a balanced diet should be the foundation, some supplements can support weight loss and kettlebell training performance.

- **Useful supplements for kettlebell training:**

Chapter 2: What should I do now?

To ensure the success of any diet, it is essential to commit to following it with determination. Only with the right mindset can you achieve your goals. To properly prepare, you need to assess the stage you are in before moving to the next stage in your diet journey. It may not seem obvious, but there is a process to follow.

The first stage is pre-contemplation. In this stage, you may not perceive your overweight or feel the motivation to make personal changes. Only strong external pressure could push you to seek help. However, you can easily become demoralized by seeing the situation as irremediable.

The second stage is contemplation. Here you recognize the problem of being overweight and start thinking about a solution. However, you may not be ready to adopt that solution yet. You will be left just thinking about what actions to take to make a change, without really being ready to act. You may procrastinate on implementing the solution itself.

The third stage is preparation. You finally decide to take action to address the problem of being overweight. You move from thinking to making the solution a reality. You start planning for the future in which you will be slimmer and healthier. However, at this stage, you may not be fully committed yet. You may still have doubts about the proposed solution, since it requires a significant change in lifestyle.

The fourth phase is action. You start to put into practice the actions to lose weight. You carefully select the foods you consume and start engaging in some form of exercise every day. This is the first concrete step towards achieving your desired goal.

During your weight loss journey, it is always important to set clear goals. Without well-defined goals, it is very likely that your entire diet plan will not develop as you imagined.

"If you fail to plan, you plan to fail"

To properly assess your current situation, it is important to list your eating habits, food preferences, and anything that could affect your weight loss. Also include your workout routines and other relevant information. Here are some points you might want to consider:

- Describe your current eating habits, such as the types of foods you usually eat and portion sizes.
- Mention any food preferences or dietary restrictions that might affect your food choices.
- Indicates the frequency and intensity of your current training, including the exercises you perform and the duration of your sessions.

Now, let's focus on the main reason why you want to lose weight. This could be related to an upcoming event, the arrival of summer, or even a special person. Try to identify the biggest reason that drives you to lose weight, such as:

- Your primary motivation may be to achieve a healthy weight to improve your overall health and prevent disease.
- You may want a more toned and attractive body to increase your self-esteem and self-admiration from others.
- Maybe you want to improve your daily energy and vitality to face life 's challenges with more ease and enthusiasm.

Apart from these reasons, there are many other benefits that you can get from losing weight. List all the benefits that come to your mind, for example:

- Improved cardiovascular health and reduced risk of heart disease.
- Increased self-esteem and positive body image.
- Greater endurance and better athletic performance.
- Reduce stress and improve overall mood.
- Improved rest and sleep quality .

Now it's time to set your weight loss goal specifically and realistically. Rather than setting an unrealistic goal, such as losing more than 10 pounds in just 2 weeks, it's important to be realistic in your expectations. So, let's formulate the goal appropriately:

- Goal: I want to lose XX pounds in a healthy and sustainable way within a reasonable period of time, such as XX months . (Be sure to enter a realistic goal that takes into account your health status and individual circumstances.)

Once you have defined the goal, write it in bold and let it sink into your mind. You can print the sheet with all this information and put it in a visible place, so you can see it every day. This constant reminder will help you stay focused on WHY you are trying to achieve this goal and the benefits you will get once you reach it.

Be persistent because it won't be easy to get out of your comfort zone.

If you find yourself making excuses instead of starting an effective diet, you should think about why you are not truly motivated to lose weight. You need to be able to step out of your comfort zone and follow Nike's famous slogan : "Just Do It."

A critical step is the maintenance phase. You need to maintain the momentum you gained during the action phase. If at any point you lose commitment or support , you risk reverting to the previous phases.

Therefore, the final phase is the most important of your diet, as it requires a long-term commitment. There are several methods you can use to stay committed.

First, make a list of the reasons why you started this journey. Look at the list every day to remind yourself of your goals. Eliminate negative thoughts from your mind. Avoid words like "never" or "deprivation" in your vocabulary. Instead of saying "I will never eat sweets," you can limit yourself to consuming them "occasionally and in moderation." Similarly, you can replace the word "deprivation" with "choice," as you choose to avoid chocolate cakes.

Visualize in your mind your future slim self doing all the things you have always wanted to do. This visualization will strengthen your motivation to follow this plan and give you the determination to succeed . Practice this visualization every day, first thing in the morning and any time during the day you feel your determination wavering.

Who to turn to when you want to lose weight?

Now that you have decided that you want to lose weight, it is important to involve other people in your weight loss journey. These people can provide you with help in various aspects, such as choosing a diet plan, identifying goals, and providing support along the way.

A Nutritionist: A nutritionist is a person with extensive knowledge who can help you understand your body and create a personalized meal plan that meets your specific needs. Remember that in most states and countries, a medical license is required to practice as a nutritionist.

A cheaper alternative to a nutritionist is a meal planner. A meal planner is an innovative, patent-pending system that acts as your own personal nutritionist or dietitian, helping you create completely balanced diets using the foods you love.

A Personal Trainer: Most people have never learned how to exercise properly. It is important, especially if you have never worked with weights, to acquire the necessary knowledge. It is not advisable to commit to a long-term contract with a personal trainer without first making sure that they understand your goals and can help you achieve them.

Friends and Family: It can be difficult to talk about your diet with others. However, there is a strategy that can make it easier for you to do so. During special occasions like parties or holidays, if someone asks , you can simply say that you are trying to eat healthier without going into the details of previous diets. This psychological approach can work to motivate you and overcome any worries or judgments.

It's OK to Fail: It's inevitable that at some point in your weight loss journey, you'll have to stumble. The key is to not give up when things get tough, but to persevere and learn from the situation.

"When the going gets tough, the tough get going."

Accept failures as part of the process and develop a resilient mindset to deal with them. If you make mistakes in your diet or miss a workout, don't stress about it. Instead, focus on your positive progress, not the small setbacks. Remember that your goal is to live a healthy lifestyle, and the good days will soon outweigh the bad days. Treat mistakes as learning opportunities and move forward. Don't let one bad day turn into a losing week or month.

A Support System: Adding some accountability to your weight loss journey can be extremely helpful. Finding a friend to share your weight loss goal with can be a great motivator. You'll feel more accountable for reaching your goals when you share them with someone who can understand the challenges you're facing. You will be able to celebrate your progress together and support each other in difficult times.

If you exercise regularly, having a friend as a workout buddy can be very valuable. They can turn a boring walk or jog into a fun and rewarding experience. Lifting weights can also be more motivating and rewarding when done with a friend, as you can encourage each other and provide hands-on support during your workouts.

If you can't find a weight loss buddy in your group of friends, don't worry. You can seek support online by joining weight loss forums or blogs.

Ultimately, working with a friend or support system can provide motivation, support, and accountability, all of which are critical to weight loss success. So, find your weight loss buddy today!

Maintaining a daily schedule is essential to your success in achieving your weight loss goals. Find a time that works best for you, whether it's early in the morning, in the afternoon, or in the evening. The important thing is to create a routine that is achievable and that allows you to set aside regular time for exercise.

Keeping a log of your activities can be very helpful. You can write down your workouts, meals, and any deviations from your schedule. If you miss a scheduled workout or have an extra snack, make a note of it and commit to doing better next time. Recording everything in a journal or on your smartphone will help you stay on track and accountable.

Knowing in advance what you need to do each day, both in terms of workouts and meals, will help you organize your day around those goals. This way, you can schedule other activities around your workout schedule and make sure you don't skip workouts.

Consistency in maintaining a daily schedule will help you achieve better results in the long run. If you frequently skip workouts or follow your diet in a haphazard manner, you may find it difficult to lose weight consistently.

Remember, the important thing is to take action, regardless of what time you decide to work out. It doesn't matter if you prefer to get up early in the morning like me or if you have other time preferences. The important thing is to do what works for you and commit to following your program consistently.

Finally, involving others in your weight loss journey can provide valuable resources and support. Working with a dietitian or nutritionist can help you create a personalized meal plan. A personal trainer can teach you proper exercise techniques and help you reach your goals. Involving friends and family can provide emotional and motivational support. Additionally, keeping a daily schedule and logging your activities will help you stay accountable and achieve lasting results. Remember that weight loss takes commitment and perseverance, but with the right support and mindset, you can reach your goals.

Chapter 3: Optimal Nutrition and Body Transformation with Kettlebells

You've probably heard many people say that a balanced diet is the key to a healthy body, but it's crucial to understand what optimal nutrition really means and why it plays such a crucial role in transforming your physique. Let's define nutrition in the context of modern fitness.

"Nutrition is the process by which we provide our bodies with all the essential elements needed for proper growth, effective fat loss, and optimal muscle development."

This updated definition emphasizes the importance of consuming the right foods that are rich in basic nutrients, especially when embarking on a kettlebell transformation journey. Strategic nutrition can not only make our bodies strong and healthy, but also enhance training results, accelerate muscle recovery, and optimize body composition. On the other hand, an inadequate nutrition plan can compromise progress, increase the risk of injury, and slow down the metabolism.

Smart Calories: The New Fitness Paradigm In 2024, the "calories in, calories out" approach has undergone a revolution. Researchers have discovered that not all calories are created equal when it comes to burning fat and building muscle, especially when combined with kettlebell training.

New nutritional science has revealed that meal timing, macronutrient composition, and food quality play a crucial role in fat burning. Kettlebell training, in particular, requires a specific nutritional strategy to maximize results.

Here's the revolutionary truth: While there are no magic pills, kettlebell training combined with targeted nutrition can dramatically accelerate fat loss and muscle definition. The goal is to create an optimal metabolic environment through nutrition and leverage the EPOC (Excess Post-exercise Oxygen Consumption) effect kettlebells generate to burn fat 24/7.

Calculating Energy Needs for Kettlebell Training In 2024, the formulas for calculating calorie needs have been updated to account for the unique impact of kettlebell training:

For men: TDEE = (10 x weight in kg + 6.25 x height in cm - 5 x age + 5) x Kettlebell Activity Factor For women: TDEE = (10 x weight in kg + 6.25 x height in cm - 5 x age - 161) x Kettlebell Activity Factor

Where the Kettlebell Activity Factor is: 1.3 for beginners (1-2 sessions/week) 1.5 for intermediates (3-4 sessions/week) 1.7 for advanced (5+ sessions/week)

This advanced formula takes into account the prolonged thermic effect of kettlebell training, allowing for more precise nutritional planning for fat loss and muscle growth.

Cyclical Nutrition to Maximize Results The latest research has shown that a cyclical nutrition strategy, combined with kettlebell training, can lead to superior results in fat loss and muscle maintenance.

The cyclical nutrition protocol includes:

- High-carb days: Coinciding with your most intense kettlebell workouts
- Low-carb load days: To optimize insulin sensitivity and promote fat burning
- Intermittent Fasting Days: To Boost Autophagy and Speed Up Metabolism

This strategy, combined with functional kettlebell training, has been shown to increase fat loss by 32 percent compared to traditional diets, according to a 2024 study published in the Journal of Functional Fitness and Nutrition.

Superfoods to Enhance Kettlebell Training In 2024, some superfoods have proven to be particularly effective in supporting kettlebell training and accelerating fat loss:

- **Goji Berries : Rich in antioxidants, they support** muscle recovery
- **Spirulina : complete protein source, promotes post-** workout protein synthesis
- **MCT Oil : Provides quick energy and promotes ketosis, ideal for high** intensity workouts
- **Turmeric : powerful anti-inflammatory, reduces post-** workout muscle soreness

- **Ashwagandha** : Adaptogen that reduces cortisol and improves performance

Incorporating these superfoods into your diet can significantly boost your kettlebell training results by accelerating fat loss and improving recovery.

The Synergy of Nutrition and Kettlebells The key to a successful body transformation in 2024 lies in the synergy of strategic nutrition and functional kettlebell training. It's no longer just about calories, but about optimizing every aspect of your diet to support the intense metabolic work that kettlebells generate.

Fat loss is a science, not a mystery. With the right nutritional strategies and a well-structured kettlebell training program, you can revolutionize your body and achieve results you once thought impossible.

Fuel your body intelligently, lift kettlebells with passion, and watch your physique transform day after day .

Eating Clean and Healthy: The Key to Transforming Your Physique

The concept of calories in and calories out remains the foundation of effective weight loss. However, the quality of calories consumed plays a crucial role in the body transformation process, especially when combined with kettlebell training.

What is "clean" eating?

The term "clean eating" refers to: "Eating whole, nutritious, minimally processed foods while avoiding ultra-processed foods and refined sugars."

This dietary approach, combined with kettlebell training, can significantly boost your fat loss and muscle toning results.

Guidelines for a clean and functional diet for kettlebell training

- **Read labels carefully** : Analyze the nutritional information and the list of ingredients of each product. Look for foods with few ingredients, all recognizable.

- **Protein Powder** : Supports muscle growth and recovery.
- **Creatine** : May improve strength and endurance during intense workouts.
- **Omega-3 fatty acids** : Reduce inflammation and support cardiovascular health.

Remember, there is no quick fix or magic pill to lose weight. The key to success is to adopt a holistic approach that combines effective kettlebell training, balanced nutrition, and a positive mindset. Educate yourself, be critical of unrealistic promises, and focus on long-term, sustainable changes. With dedication, patience, and the right strategies, you can revolutionize your body and achieve your fitness goals in a healthy and lasting way.

Conclusion

Ultimately, losing weight in a healthy and sustainable way requires a comprehensive approach that goes beyond simply counting calories. It requires an understanding of your body, your habits, and your environment. With the right tools, the right support, and a resilient mindset, you can achieve and maintain a healthy weight for the long haul. Always remember to consult a healthcare professional before starting any new diet or exercise program, especially if you have pre-existing health conditions."

- **Go Whole Grains** : Opt for brown rice, quinoa, oats , and 100% whole grain bread. These provide sustained energy for intense kettlebell workouts.
- **Load up on fruits and vegetables** : Aim to fill half your plate with colorful vegetables, and vary them often. Fruits and vegetables provide essential vitamins, minerals, and antioxidants for post-workout recovery .
- **Cooking at Home** : Preparing your own meals gives you complete control over the ingredients. Try to prepare balanced meals for the week ahead of time, including protein snacks for pre- and post-kettlebell workouts.
- **Choose Lean Protein** : Chicken , turkey, fish, legumes, and eggs are great sources of protein to support the muscle growth that kettlebell exercises stimulate. Aim to include protein in every main meal .
- **Avoid processed meats** : Deli meats, sausages, and other processed meats are high in sodium and saturated fat. Opt for lean cuts of fresh meat.
- **Smart Snacks** : Replace low-nutrient snacks with unsalted nuts, seeds, fresh fruit, or Greek yogurt . These provide quality energy to power through your workout sessions.
- **Hydration** : Drink plenty of water throughout the day, especially before, during and after kettlebell workouts to maintain optimal performance.
- **Flexibility** : Allow yourself the occasional controlled "cheat." A long-term sustainable diet is one that doesn't leave you feeling deprived.

Strategy for Eating Healthy Out

Eating out can be a challenge, but many restaurants today offer healthy options:

- Choose salads rich in vegetables with added protein (grilled chicken, salmon, tofu).
- Opt for dishes with a good source of lean protein and steamed or grilled vegetables.
- Ask for condiments and sauces separately to control the quantity.
- Avoid fried or cheese-rich dishes, preferring cooking methods such as grilling or steaming.

Integrating Clean Eating with Kettlebell Training

- **Pre-workout** : Eat a light meal rich in complex carbohydrates and lean protein about 1-2 hours before your workout. Example: Whole wheat toast with avocado and egg.
- **Post-workout** : Within 30 minutes of finishing your session, consume a combination of protein and carbohydrates to aid recovery. Example: Whey Protein Shake with Banana and Spinach.
- **Main Meals** : Balance your plate with 1/4 lean protein, 1/4 complex carbohydrates, and 1/2 colorful vegetables.
- **Meal timing** : Spread your calorie intake throughout the day into 3 main meals and 2-3 snacks, keeping your energy level stable.
- Benefits of Clean Eating Combined with Kettlebell Training
- **Metabolism Booster** : Combining clean eating and high intensity kettlebell training boosts your metabolism, increasing calorie expenditure even at rest.
- **Improved body composition** : Reduced body fat and increased lean muscle mass.
- **Increased Energy** : Whole, unprocessed foods provide consistent energy, improving performance during workouts.
- **Optimized Recovery** : A nutrient-rich diet supports muscle repair and reduces post-workout inflammation.
- **Improved overall health** : Reduced risk of chronic disease and boosted immune system.

Embracing clean eating is not just a weight loss strategy, but a holistic approach to improving your health, athletic performance, and quality of life. Combined with a well-structured kettlebell training program, it is a powerful synergy to transform your body.

Change doesn't happen overnight. Start with small, sustainable changes and gradually build new habits. Consistency in clean eating and kettlebell training will yield amazing results over time.

Water: Your Secret Fat Burning Ally

The latest research has confirmed that proper hydration is key to optimizing your kettlebell workout results and boosting your metabolism. While the traditional recommendation of drinking 8 glasses of water a day still stands, experts are now suggesting a more personalized approach based on body weight and activity intensity.

To determine your daily fluid requirement, use this updated formula: multiply your weight in kg by 0.033. For example, a person weighing 80 kg should aim to consume approximately 2.64 liters of water per day. However, when incorporating intense kettlebell training, you should increase this amount by 20-30% to compensate for fluid loss through sweating.

Why is hydration crucial for burning fat with kettlebells?

- Enhance Performance: Water optimizes muscle function and endurance during high-intensity kettlebell exercises, allowing you to push longer and burn more calories.
- Boosts Metabolism: Recent studies have shown that drinking 16 ounces of water can increase your resting metabolism by up to 30% for an hour, amplifying the fat-burning effects of your kettlebell workout.
- Supports Muscle Recovery: Proper hydration reduces post-workout inflammation and accelerates tissue repair, allowing you to get back to the gym faster.
- Enhances Thermogenesis: Cold water forces the body to burn extra calories to warm it, further increasing energy expenditure.
- Control Appetite: Drinking water before meals can reduce calorie intake by up to 13%, supporting your weight loss goals.

Hydration Strategies to Maximize Kettlebell Results:

- Pre-Hydration: Drink 500ml of water 30 minutes before your kettlebell workout to prepare your body for the intensity to come.
- Hydration During Workout: Sip 5-8 ounces of water every 15-20 minutes of kettlebell exercise to maintain optimal performance.

- Post-workout rehydration: Consume 500ml of water within 30 minutes of finishing your session to accelerate recovery and protein synthesis.
- Naturally Flavored Water: Add slices of lemon, cucumber or mint to your water to make it more palatable and benefit from its antioxidant properties.
- Smart Tracking: Use hydration tracking apps or smart water bottles to make sure you hit your daily water goals.

In addition to listening to experts, it is essential to develop an awareness of your body. Thirst is a reliable indicator of the need for hydration, but when you are doing an intense kettlebell workout, it is essential to anticipate this signal. Considering the high intensity of kettlebell exercises, always keeping a bottle of water on hand becomes crucial, especially during more intense sessions or in hot environments.

Water is the essential fuel for your kettlebell transformation. Not only is it calorie-free, it amplifies the fat-burning effects of your workout, improves performance, and speeds recovery. Gradually replacing sugary drinks with water at mealtimes will not only reduce your calorie intake, but it will also optimize your body composition, allowing you to maximize the weight-loss and muscle-toning benefits of kettlebells.

Every sip of water brings you closer to your goal of burning fat and building a sculpted kettlebell physique. Start implementing these hydration strategies today and prepare to see amazing results in your physical transformation!

Chapter 4: The Importance of Exercise

In this chapter I will reveal to you the most effective method to melt fat like butter on a boiling pan.

Exercise:

First of all, the human body is designed to move, period. In addition to the obvious benefits of maintaining a healthy body weight, exercise offers numerous other benefits that go beyond aesthetics:

- Fight diseases such as stroke, diabetes and heart disease
- Improve mood and reduce stress
- Increase energy levels throughout the day
- Promote quality sleep and regulate your sleep cycle
- Improve your sex life, increase your self- confidence

"A recent survey found that seven in ten adults do not exercise regularly, and nearly four in ten are not physically active." This lack of physical activity is closely linked to a higher risk of chronic disease and premature death, with approximately 300,000 deaths a year linked to inactivity.

Before you start: Consult a doctor

Before starting any exercise program, especially if you have been inactive for a long time, it is essential to consult a doctor. This is especially true if you are new to exercise or have pre-existing health conditions. A medical check-up will help you prevent injuries and establish a safe and effective exercise plan.

Fat Loss Myths: Why Running Isn't Always the Best Solution

When it comes to fat loss, people often think of aerobic exercise, such as running, as the key to fast results. While it's true that running increases your heart rate and helps improve cardiovascular endurance, the myth that it's the most effective exercise for burning fat is misleading.

Recent studies show that once your body gets used to running training, progress tends to slow down. According to research by Peele (2010), the body becomes more efficient at performing the exercise, burning fewer calories over time. In other words, your effort remains the same, but the fat-burning benefits decrease.

The Solution: Kettlebell – The Most Effective Fat Burning Workout

On the contrary, using kettlebells has proven to be one of the most powerful techniques for efficiently burning fat and transforming the body. This type of training not only improves strength, but also combines resistance and cardiovascular exercises in one session, making it much more productive than running.

Why are kettlebells up to 3,000% more efficient at burning fat than running?

High-Intensity Interval Training (HIIT): Using kettlebells pushes your body to a much higher level of intensity than running steadily. Kettlebell training involves short bursts of energy followed by short periods of rest, which boosts your metabolism and promotes fat burning hours after your workout.

1. **Engagement of multiple muscle groups** : Unlike running, which focuses primarily on the leg muscles, kettlebells activate all the major muscle groups: arms, shoulders, abs, back and legs, allowing you to burn more calories in less time.
2. **Increased Metabolism** : Kettlebell exercises promote the afterburn phenomenon, also known as post-exercise oxygen consumption (EPOC). This means you will continue to burn calories even after you have finished your workout.
3. **Exercise Variety** : Kettlebell training is versatile and dynamic. You can switch between strength and cardiovascular exercises in a single session, keeping your body constantly engaged and preventing boredom and stagnation.

Kettlebell Benefits: Your Ally for a Toned Body

Kettlebell training is not only effective for fat loss, but it also has many other benefits:

- muscle strength and endurance
- Increases flexibility and joint mobility
- Develops coordination and balance
- Burns more calories in less time than traditional aerobic exercises

Incorporating kettlebells into your routine allows you to see visible results in less time, improving your body composition and accelerating fat loss.

If you're tired of seeing little progress with your running and are looking for a more efficient way to lose fat and tone your body, kettlebell training is the answer. With the right combination of high-intensity exercises, you can finally unlock your body's potential and achieve lasting results.

Why is HIIT better than running?

When it comes to burning fat and sculpting your body, there is nothing more effective than **HIIT** (High-Intensity Interval Training). This innovative approach not only drastically reduces the duration of training sessions, but it can burn up to **9 times more fat** than traditional running (Cossaboon). In other words, it is up to **36 times more effective** , while requiring only a fraction of the time!

But how exactly does it work? The intensity of HIIT is key. During each session, you burn significantly more calories than other types of training. Although a smaller portion of the calories burned come directly from fat, the **overall calorie count** is significantly higher, resulting in **greater weight loss** and an overall benefit for the body. This is ideal for those who want to maximize results in a short amount of time.

The post-workout effect: burn fat for 24 hours!

One of the most incredible benefits of **HIIT** is the "afterburn" effect or **EPOC** (Excess Post-Exercise Oxygen Consumption). After you finish your high-intensity workout, your **metabolism stays up for 24 hours** , which means you continue to burn calories, even while you're relaxing on the couch in the evening! This phenomenon is not as present in traditional running or longer but less intense workouts.

Kettlebell Workouts: The Perfect Combination With HIIT

If you want **to revolutionize your body and burn fat even more efficiently, try combining HIIT with kettlebell** exercises . Kettlebells not only increase strength, but also improve endurance and **cardiovascular conditioning** , further accelerating the fat burning process. The dynamic movements that characterize this tool involve multiple muscle groups, making the workout more intense and complete.

One of the reasons kettlebells are so powerful is their ability to work the **core, leg and arm** muscles simultaneously , combining aerobic and anaerobic training in a single session. The result? **Greater strength and a toned body in less time. This type of** high- intensity training , combined with targeted exercises with kettlebells, is an optimal solution for those who want **to burn fat quickly** , improve body composition and obtain visible results in just a few weeks.

How often should you train?

You don't have to work out every day to see significant results. With HIIT and kettlebells, just **3 sessions a week** of about 20-30 minutes are enough to start noticing a transformation in your body. This makes HIIT perfect for those who are short on time, but still want to get a **sculpted body and burn fat quickly** .

If you want **to burn fat** , tone your body and maximize your results without spending hours in the gym, HIIT **combined with kettlebell exercises** is the best choice. Get the most out of your workout with short but intense sessions and harness the power of "afterburn" to continue burning fat even while you rest. Don't wait: start your journey to a **toned, leaner and stronger body** today!

How does HIIT work ?

High Intensity Interval Training (HIIT) uses a dual-intensity approach to achieve fast and lasting fat loss results. Unlike a traditional, constant-intensity workout,

HIIT alternates between two levels of intensity, dramatically increasing calorie burn and improving metabolism.

- **Level 1** : This is a moderate intensity level, such as a brisk jog or riding a stationary bike.
- **Level 2** : This is a high intensity level, such as a sprint at maximum speed or explosion exercises, which last only a few seconds.

The classic protocol consists of working at a moderate intensity for 2-2.5 minutes, then switching to an explosive session of 10-30 seconds. This pattern is repeated for a total duration of 15-20 minutes, allowing you to make the most of the "afterburn" effect (EPOC), which stimulates the body to burn extra calories for hours after training. This way, not only will you burn fat during physical activity, but your body will continue to do so during the recovery period. The results will be seen in a short time, with a significant reduction in fat mass.

Keep your heart rate in the "good zone "

To get the most out of HIIT, it's essential to keep your heart rate high enough during peak intensity. But what's your ideal heart rate?

Calculate your maximum heart rate by subtracting your age from 220. For example, if you are 30 years old, your maximum heart rate is 190 beats per minute.

During high intensity sessions, aim to hit 85% of this number, or about 162 bpm. This will ensure you are working in the "fat burning zone" and maximizing your calorie burn.

One sign that you are working correctly is difficulty maintaining a conversation during the exercise. If you can still talk easily, you need to push yourself further. Don't be afraid to step out of your comfort zone ; this is where real physical transformations happen.

Combine Kettlebell Strength Training Into Your Routine

In addition to HIIT, kettlebell strength training is one of the most effective methods for losing weight, improving posture, and toning muscles. Unlike traditional weight lifting, using kettlebells allows you to work on strength, endurance, and mobility in a single session. Women, in particular, can benefit greatly from incorporating kettlebells into their workout routine without fear of developing a "muscular" appearance.

When done correctly, kettlebell movements stimulate lean muscle growth, resulting in a lean, toned appearance. This type of workout also improves flexibility and increases functional strength, which is very useful in everyday life. Plus, exercises like the "kettlebell swing" activate a huge amount of muscle at once, burning calories and boosting your metabolism for hours.

Resistance training prevents osteoporosis

In addition to burning fat and sculpting your body, resistance training with kettlebells has been shown to be an ally in the prevention of osteoporosis, especially in women. Studies confirm that weight training is essential for bone health, as it stimulates bone density, reducing the risk of fractures.

Kettlebell exercises can be used for both the lower body, such as squats and lunges, and the upper body, involving the shoulders, arms and core. The metabolism remains active even several hours after the workout, thanks to the energy expenditure required for muscle recovery.

Fat Burning Tool

Kettlebell training is therefore an excellent choice for anyone who wants to lose weight and tone their body. Thanks to their versatility, kettlebells allow you to combine cardiovascular training with strength training, accelerating the fat burning process and improving endurance. Even a short 20- minute workout a day can lead to visible results in just a few weeks.

The Combined Power of HIIT and Kettlebell

By combining the power of HIIT with the effectiveness of kettlebell training, you can transform your body quickly and lastingly. These two tools, together, are incredibly effective at burning fat , increasing lean muscle mass, and improving your overall fitness. Be sure to consult a doctor before starting a new workout program, especially if you have gone a long time without working out.

Why train with a kettlebell?

The first time I saw someone working out with a kettlebell, I didn't fully understand its effectiveness. But after being invited to a workout, I realized how powerful this simple yet versatile piece of equipment is for transforming your body and burning fat quickly and efficiently.

The kettlebell originated in Russia and is now an indispensable piece of equipment in the fitness world. If you have never heard of the kettlebell, it is probably because you have not yet been exposed to one of the most effective training tools available on the modern fitness market. Training with the kettlebell is a revolutionary method, which allows you to achieve maximum results in a relatively short time.

The Benefits of Kettlebell Training

If you are looking for a way to burn fat fast, gain strength and tone your body, kettlebell training is the perfect solution for you. Let's see the many benefits of this amazing tool:

- Increase functional strength and lean muscle mass: Each kettlebell exercise trains multiple muscle groups at the same time, optimizing every movement.
- Burn fat efficiently: Thanks to the intensity of your workouts, you can increase your metabolism and burn more calories even at rest.
- Reduces Body Fat: In addition to burning calories, kettlebell training is designed to dramatically reduce body fat and accelerate weight loss.
- Improve your endurance and cardio fitness: The kettlebell allows you to improve your physical endurance and cardiovascular capacity without requiring long traditional cardio training sessions.
- Strengthen your core and improve stability: Developing a strong core is essential not only for having ripped abs but also for preventing injuries and improving posture.
- Versatile and low-cost workout: You can use the kettlebell in any space, without the need for a gym membership or expensive equipment.

- Suitable for any fitness level: Whether you are a beginner or an experienced athlete, kettlebells can be easily adapted to your skill level and goals.

The Kettlebell: Suitable for Every Situation

Many of us have followed traditional training programs aimed at specific goals, such as losing weight or improving muscular endurance. However, kettlebell training prepares you for any challenge life throws your way, from weight lifting to cardiovascular endurance.

In recent years, general physical preparation (GPP) has gained popularity not only among professional athletes, but also among those who want to improve their general physical fitness. The kettlebell is one of the most effective tools for developing GPP, helping you improve strength, endurance, mobility, and agility.

Key Kettlebell Exercises

With a few basic exercises like the swing, squat, and Turkish get-up, you can achieve incredible levels of strength and definition. These movements are designed to work your entire body and improve your mobility and stability. Kettlebell training not only builds muscle, but also develops the mental toughness needed to tackle physical and everyday challenges.

Choosing the right kettlebell

If you are just starting out with kettlebells, it is important to choose the right weight to avoid injury and maximize your results. For men, it is recommended to start with a 16kg (about 35lbs) kettlebell, while for women, it is more appropriate to start with an 8-12kg (18-26lbs) kettlebell. With time and experience, you can gradually increase the weight as your strength and endurance improve.

Safety and technology: the key to success

Safety is of the essence when starting a kettlebell training program. Always consult your doctor before starting a new exercise program, especially if you have pre-existing health conditions. Perform a proper warm-up before each session and be sure to maintain proper form to avoid injury.

When performing kettlebell exercises, pay special attention to the position of your feet: they must be firmly planted on the ground. Minimalist shoes are the best option , or you can also train barefoot for greater stability.

Training and progression

If you are new to kettlebell training, it is essential to learn proper technique before increasing the intensity of your workouts. Spend the first week practicing the swing movement, the most important of the kettlebell exercises, as it will help you build a solid foundation of strength and endurance.

In the next chapter, you will find a detailed training program that will guide you step by step . Each exercise will be illustrated with images and detailed instructions to ensure correct execution and help you achieve the best results in terms of strength and muscle definition.

Kettlebell workout routine

The kettlebell training program I propose is structured over four days a week, with alternating sessions to ensure a balance between training and rest. For example, you could train on Monday and Tuesday, rest on Wednesday, and resume on Thursday and Friday. Each training session is designed to challenge the body in a complete and progressive way.

Remember, consistency is key. Stick to the program for 8 weeks, along with a balanced diet and proper rest, and you will be amazed at the results you get.

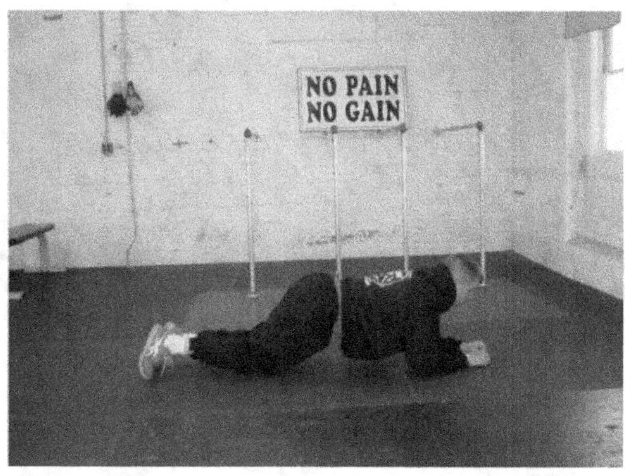

Starting position for the Front Plank

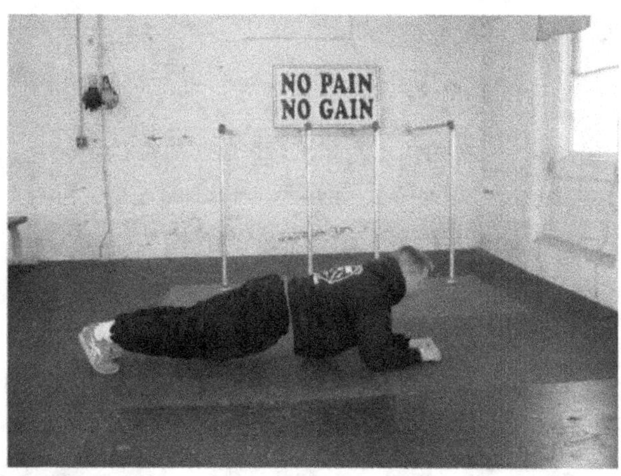

The starting position is on your hands and knees with a flat back. Contract your abdominal muscles. Without rotating your torso or bending or arching your spine, lift yourself into a push-up position with your weight on your forearms and toes. Keep your head up and looking forward. The goal is to hold this position for 60 seconds. If you can't hold for 1 minute, repeat until 1 minute has passed. Continue breathing as you perform this exercise.

HIP FLEXOR STRETCHING

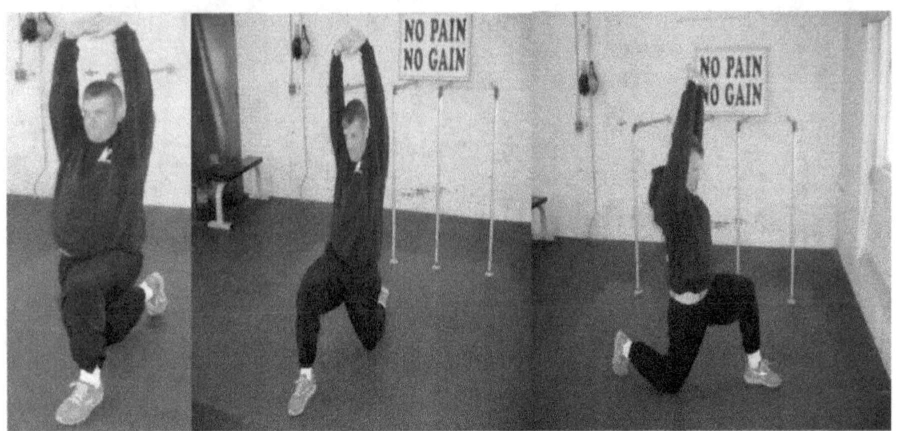

Movement :

1. Start with your left knee on the floor and your right leg raised with both arms above your head.
2. Press and hold for about 10 seconds.
3. Switch to the other side and hold for 10 seconds.

Note: This warm up exercise promotes stretching of the core, hip flexors, back, quads, lats and is just a great general stretch to loosen up. This is perhaps the best overall stretch you can do before any physical event.

PUSH-UPS

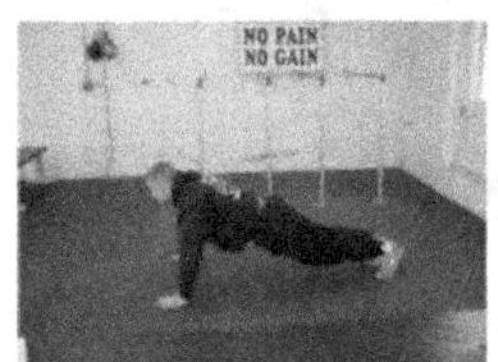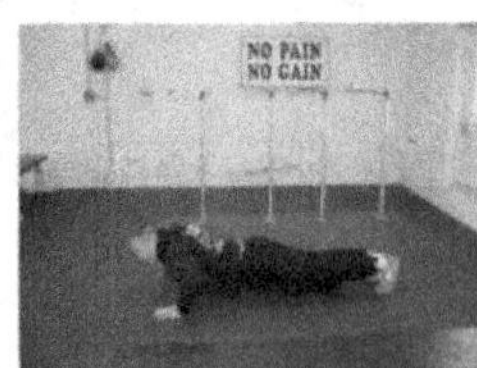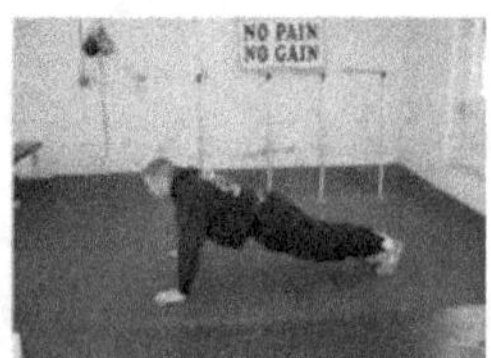

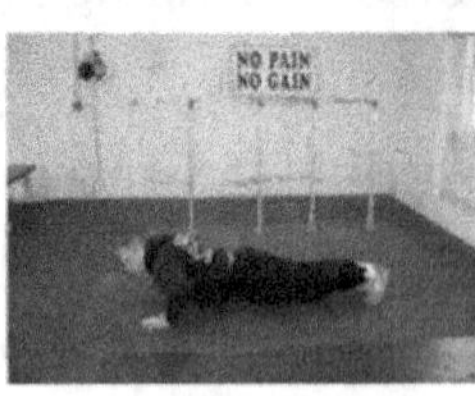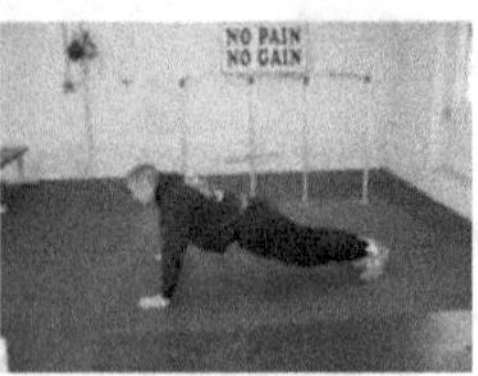

I realize that most people think they know how to do a push-up.

Movement :

Bend your elbows, lowering your body until your upper arms are parallel to the floor. Extend your arms fully so that your elbows are "locked."

The key is to fully extend in the raised position with your arms locked out. Second, make sure that when you are in the lowered position your arms

are parallel to the ground. Don't think fast here, just do them slowly and in a controlled manner for the full effect of this movement.

Variation : If you are unable to perform a push-up as illustrated, assume a kneeling position to perform them properly. This is a natural progression.

KETTLEBELL SWING

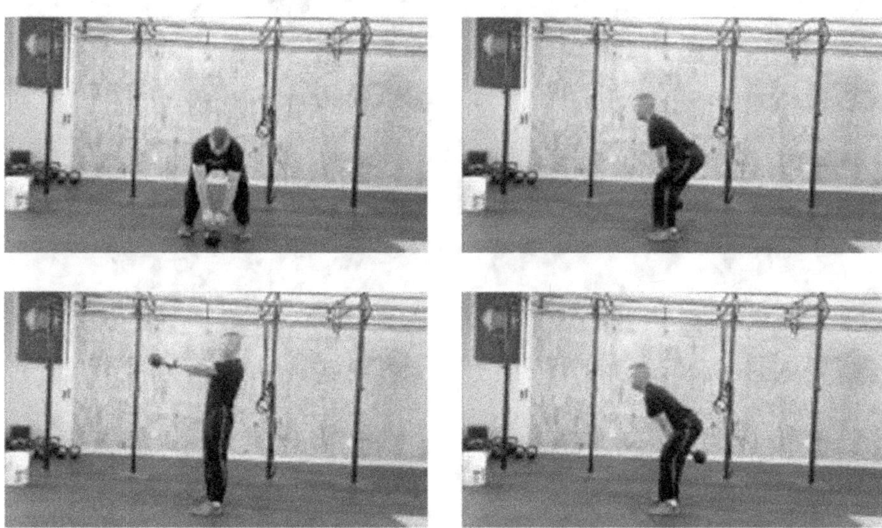

Movement:

1. Squat down with your back straight and lift the weight.
2. Don't confuse this with a vertical back, just keep it straight.
3. Don't turn your back.
4. Squat down and stand tall with your shoulders back.
5. Think about sitting rather than diving.

Make sure your hips are extended as well as your knees up with your body in a straight line. For the Russian swing shown here, the bell should never go above parallel . Make sure you are barefoot or wearing a minimalist shoe so your feet are flat.

Precautions : Work initially with a light weight until you can perform the movement correctly.

TURKISH TRAINING

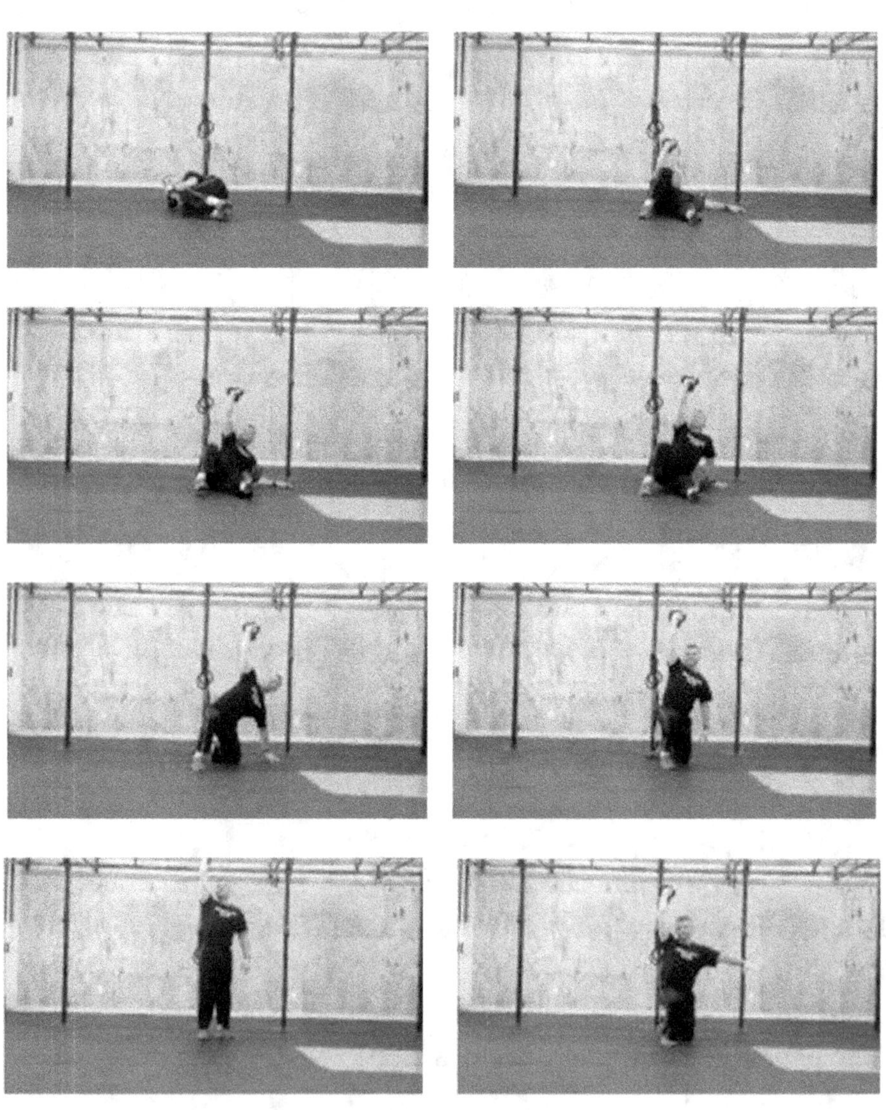

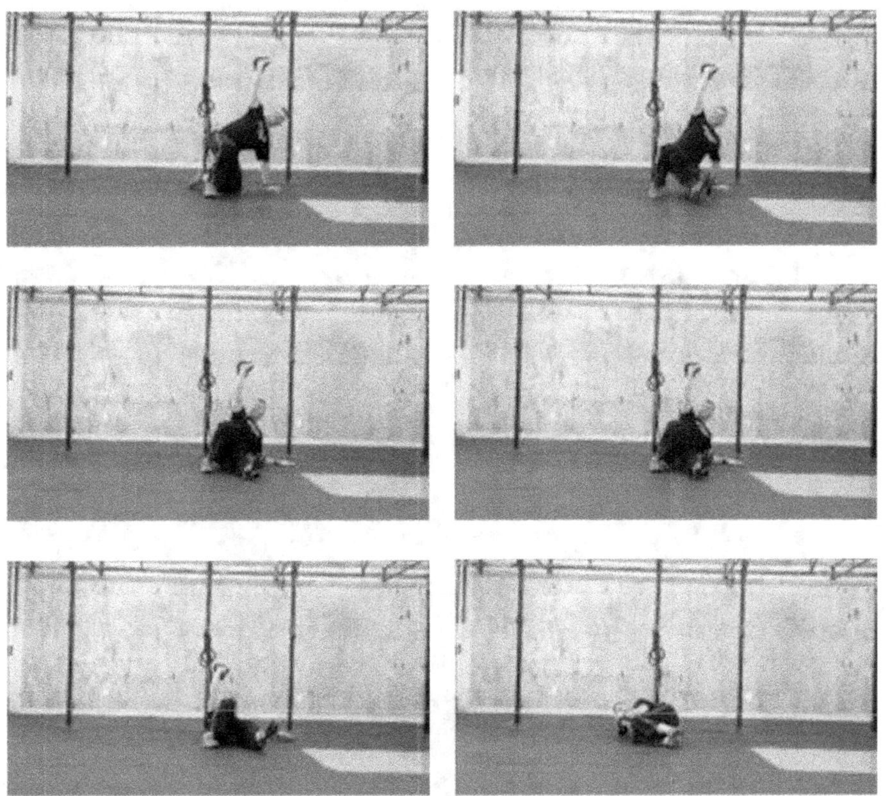

Movement : Use both hands while in the fetal position to lift the kettlebell off the ground at the beginning of the movement and at the end of the movement.

Next you want to set up your foot and hand. Notice that the arm on the side of the kettlebell is vertical with a straight wrist. The knee on the side of the kettlebell is bent to prepare you to eventually stand up. Both your lats and core are engaged and ready to work. The arm opposite the kettlebell is positioned at 45 degrees and the opposite leg is straight.

Lock your elbow and keep it locked throughout the movement.

Always keep your shoulder in a "packed" position throughout the movement.

Rise up gently and slowly and concentrate on each position.

This is not a quick exercise.

Caution : This looks deceptively easy. Use a very light weight (10 pounds) or even a sneaker until you get to each position.

Break

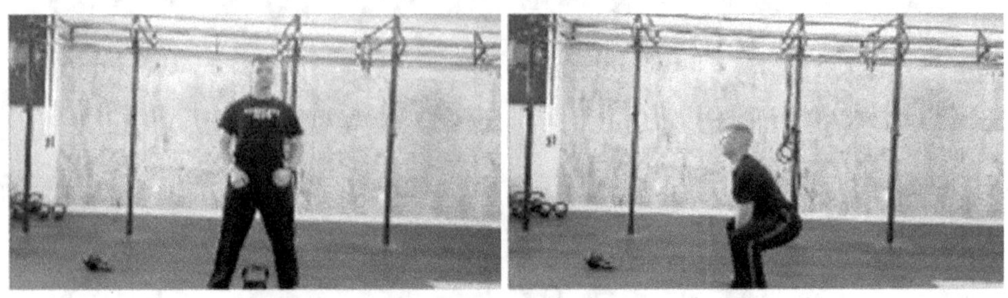

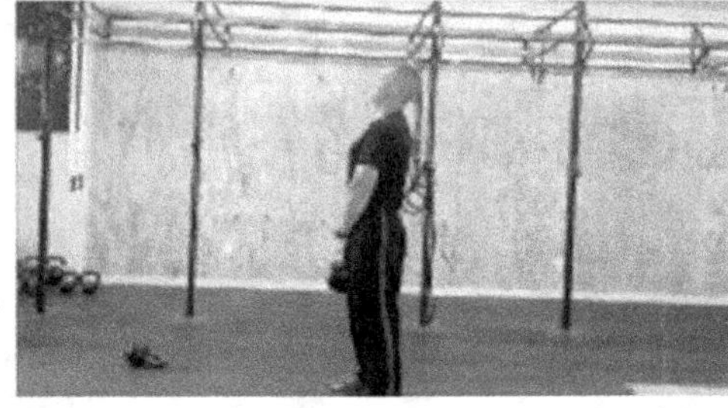

Movement :

Straddle the bell with your feet slightly wider than shoulder-width apart.

Squat down with your arms straight down between your legs and grasp the bell handle with both hands. Make sure your shoulders are over the bell and keep your back straight. Pull the bell off the floor by extending your hips and knees making sure your chest is lifted. Lower the kettlebell as you squat and keep your back straight with a vertical spine.

Precaution : Make sure you do not round your back. Make sure you can properly perform an air squat without weight before adding any weight.

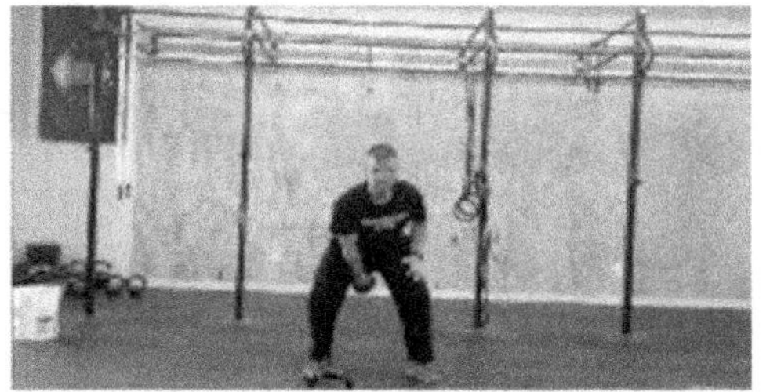 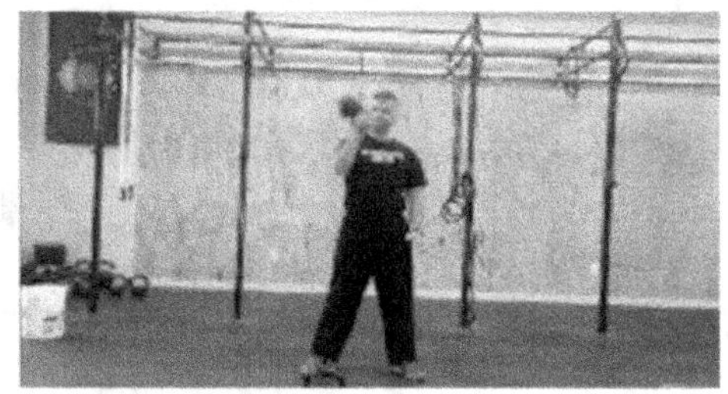

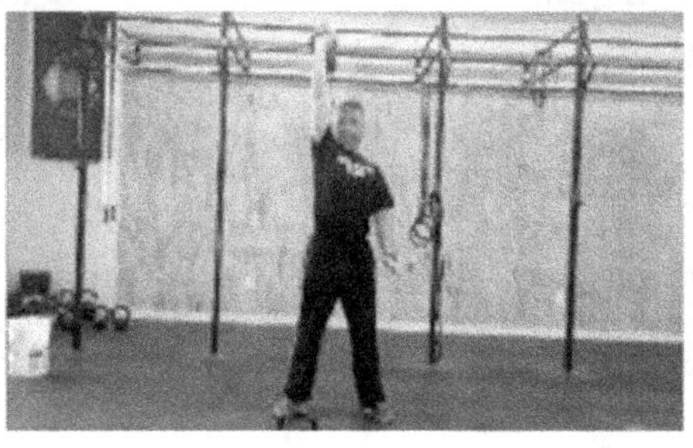

Movement :

1. Start with Russian style swing.
2. Grip the bell gently without "slamming" the bell onto your wrist.
3. You can do this by "punching" at the top of the movement.
4. When you block high, your arm should be at head height.
5. Lower the bell to complete one swing and repeat as necessary.

Precaution : Keep your back straight, work with a weight you can safely control.

Learn the Rack: I was shown this by a trainer about 5 years ago when I first started using kettlebells. I suggest you practice it so you learn the move. It will help with the Rack and Clean.

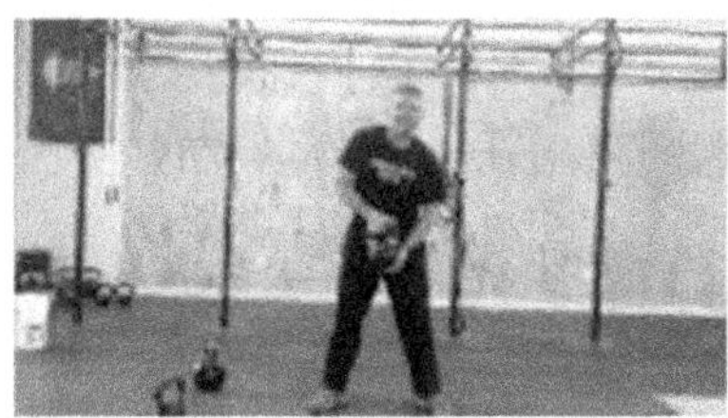 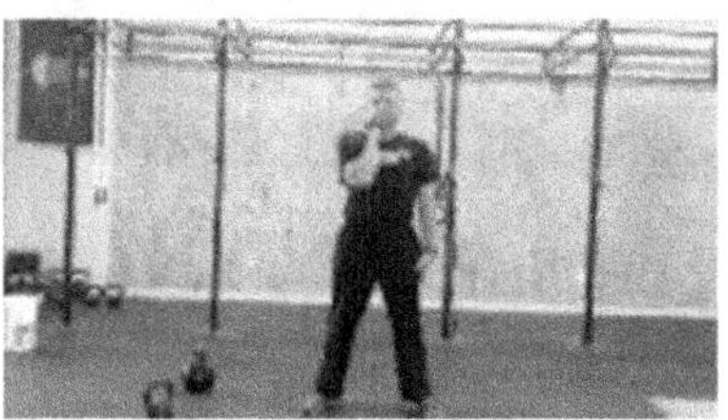

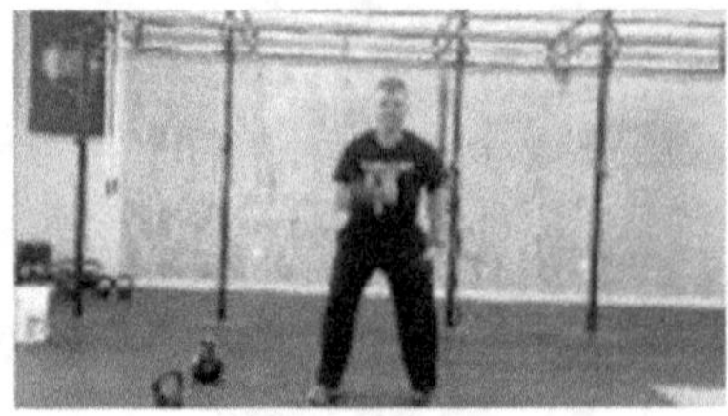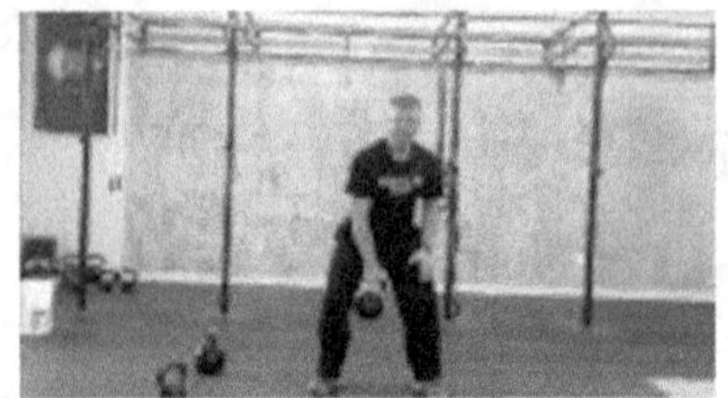

Movement :

1. Lift the bell with one hand
2. Use your second hand to position the bell
3. Now you are in the rack position or where the clean ends
4. Lower the kettlebell by moving your hips back and "sitting down"

The bell moves completely vertically downward by moving the hips back and not pushing the bell forward

Precaution : Keep your back straight, use a lighter weight until you learn the movement.

THE RACK

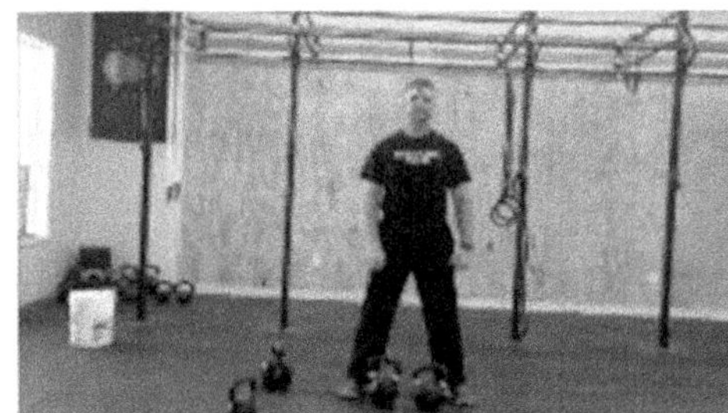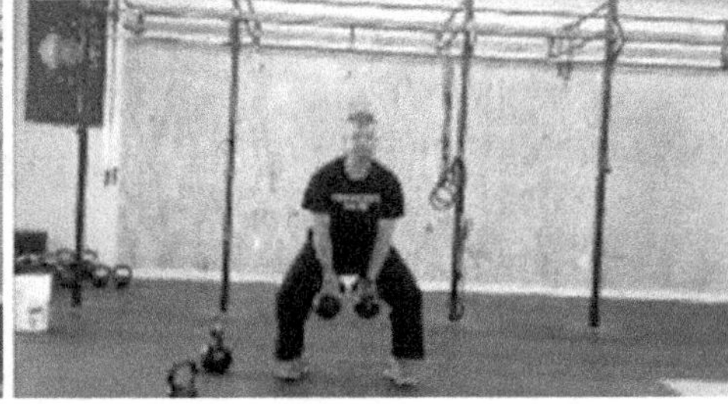

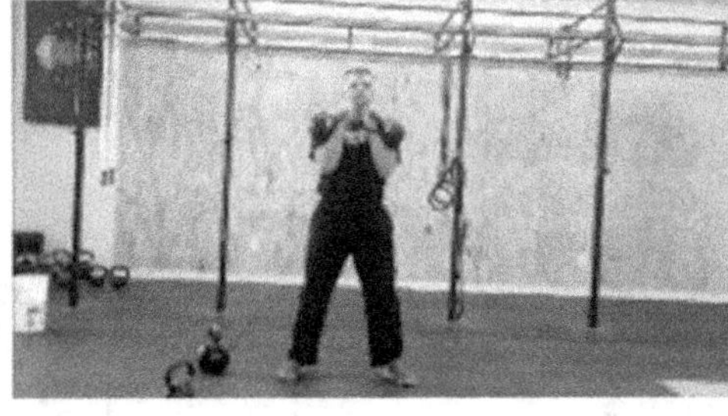

Movement :

1. Position yourself on top of the kettlebells.

2. Take a deep breath and hold and pull back between your legs.
3. As the kettlebells come back (inhale), bend your knees slightly, pushing your hips back allowing the kettlebells to pass between your legs.
4. Make sure your back is straight.
5. Using your glutes like a rubber band, open your hips and push the kettlebell forward. As you drive with your hips (exhale) until you reach a triple extension.
6. The bells should land between your arms and forearms, with your elbow bent during the movement. Your bells are now in a racked position.

Precaution : Make sure your back is straight and select a weight that is within your ability to lift safely.

Double front squat with kettlebell

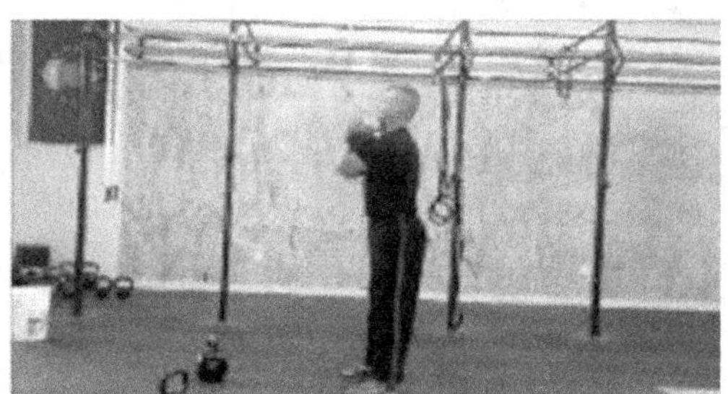
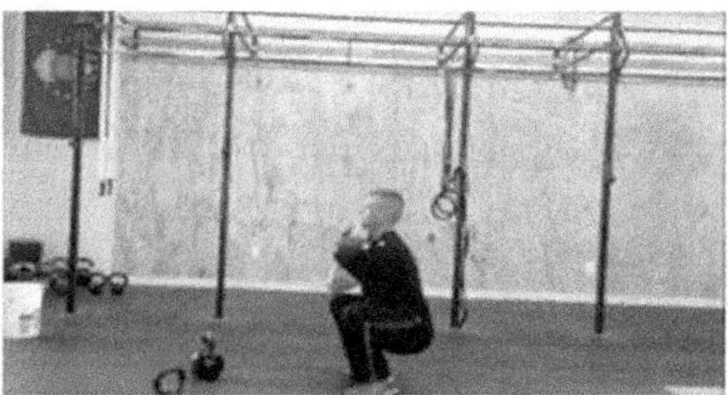

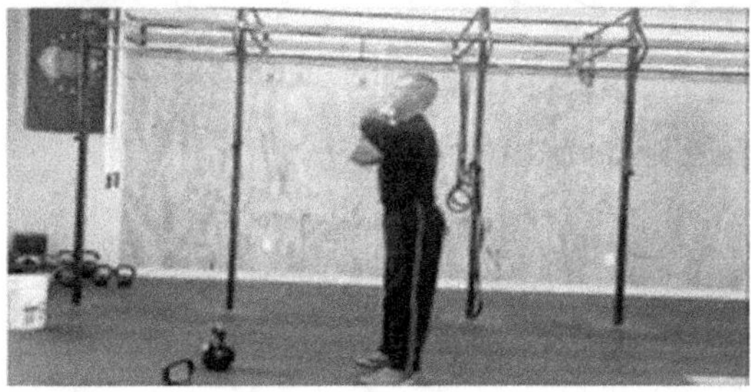

Movement :

1. Start with the bells in the rack position.
2. Place the handles just above your collarbone.
3. Keep your feet a little wider than shoulder-width apart.
4. Inhale as you sit down, keeping your back straight.
5. Exhale as you rise and stand up.

Precautions : Do not turn your back. Make sure your back is straight. Select a weight that you can move safely.

CLEAN

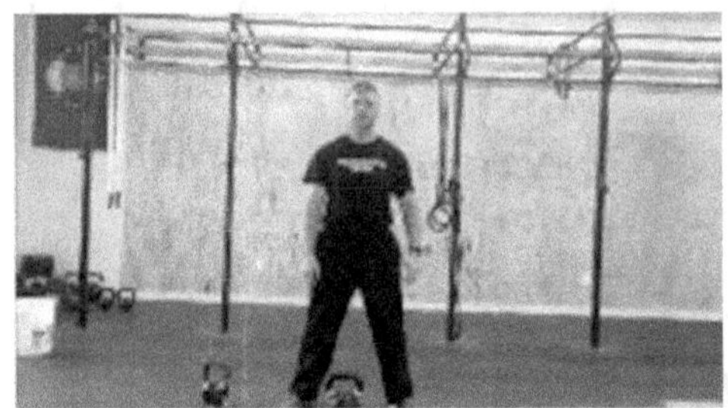 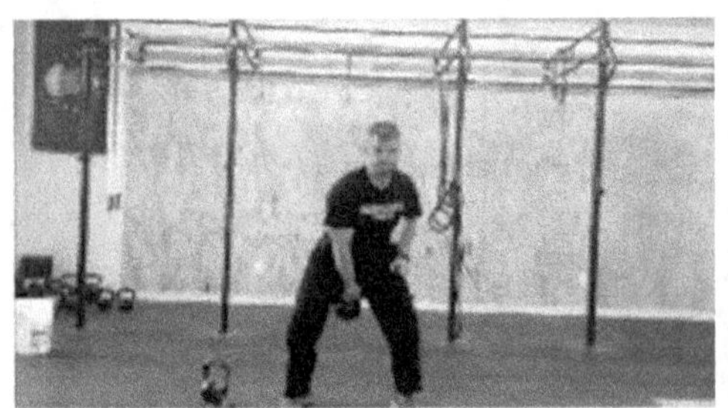

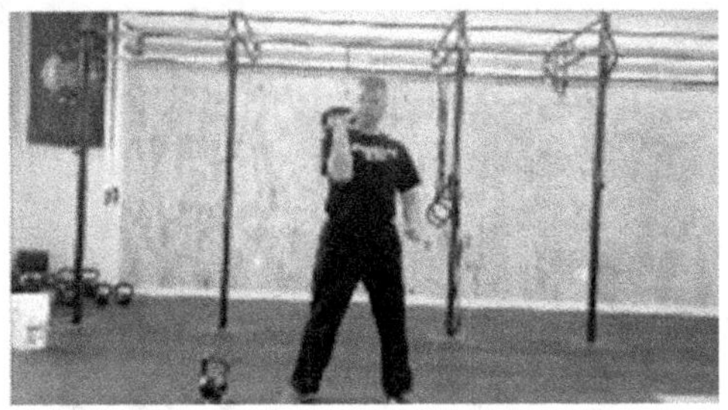

Movement :

1. Straddle the kettlebell with your feet slightly wider than shoulder-width apart.
2. The elbow should be part of the torso.
3. Your hips will do all the work.
4. Make the bell travel in a straight line; which is the shortest distance between 2 objects.
5. Do not lower your knees when receiving or "transferring" the bell.
6. Avoid banging your wrist or forearm.

Precautions : Keep your back straight and choose a weight you can work with safely.

PRESS

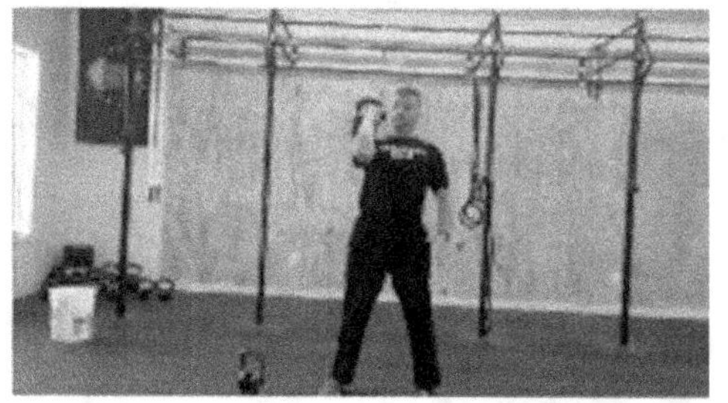 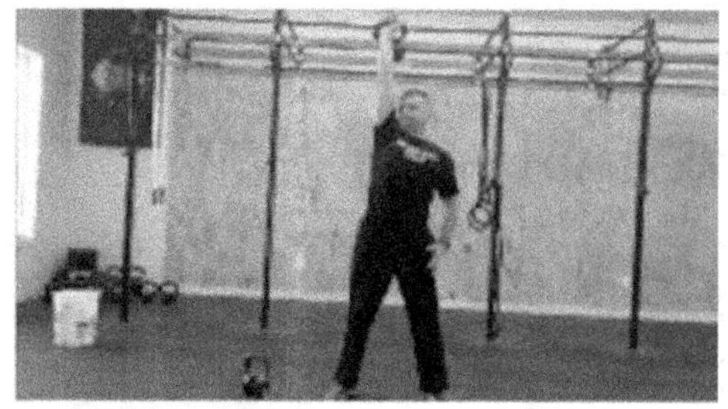

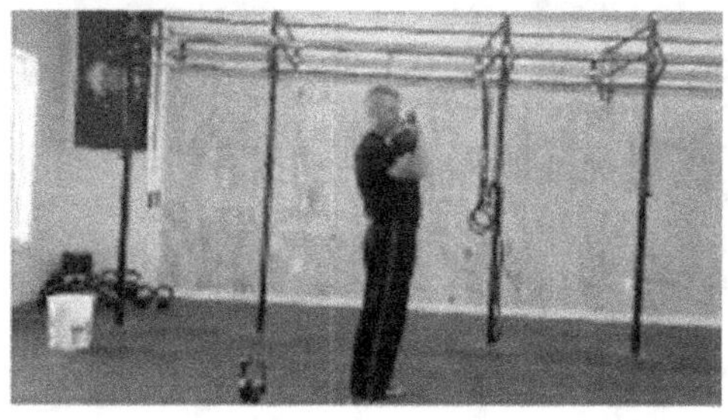

Movement :

1. Stand with your feet slightly wider than shoulder-width apart.
2. Take the bell from the rack or clean it off the floor and place it in front of your chest with the bell against the outside of your arm.
3. Push the bell up until your arm is fully extended above your head.
4. Lower yourself in front of your chest.

Precaution : Make sure you use a weight that allows you to perform the movement correctly.

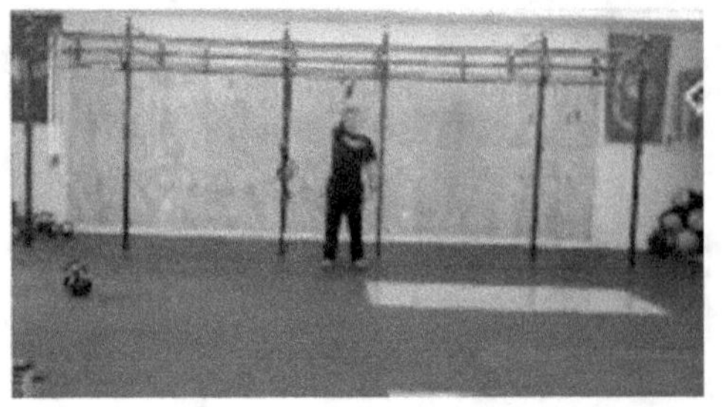 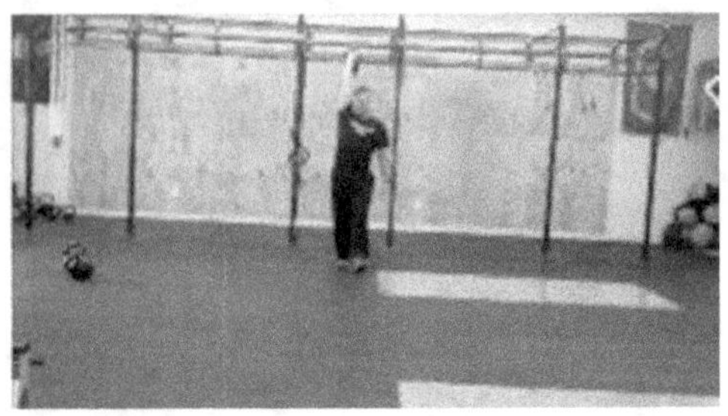

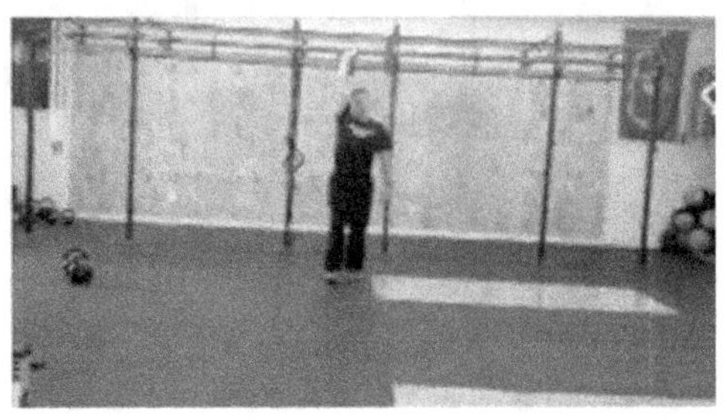

Overhead or Waiters Walk

Movement :

1. Start with the kettlebell in the press out position.
2. Make sure your shoulder and elbow are in a "locked" position.
3. Start walking.

Precautions : Make sure you have a clear path (of course), select your weight carefully.

Suitcase Carry

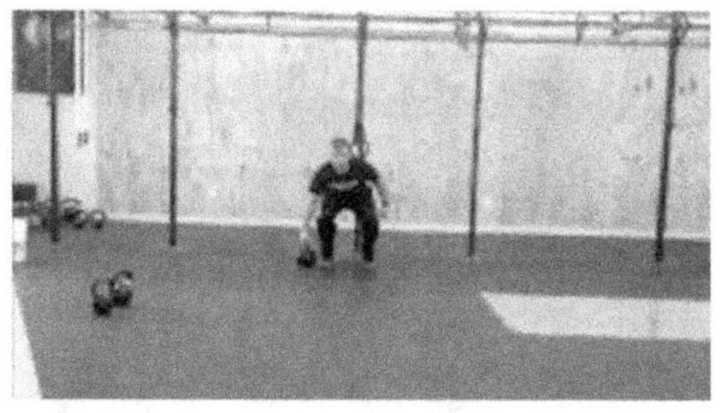 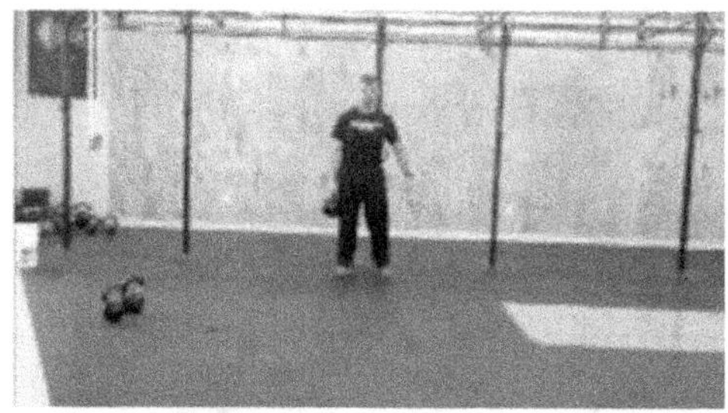

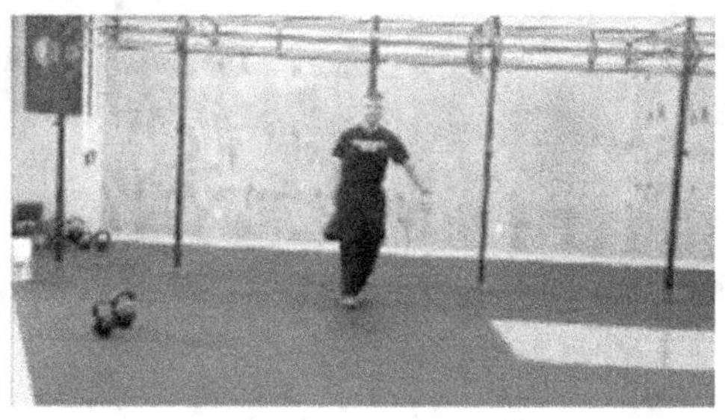

Movement :

1. Lift the bell as you would a suitcase lift before transporting.
2. Keep your shoulders level and core tight without compensating from side to side.
3. You may need more weight to achieve the desired effect.

Precautions : Make sure your back is straight and not rounded when lifting or putting down the weight. As always, select a weight that you can move safely.

Rack Walk

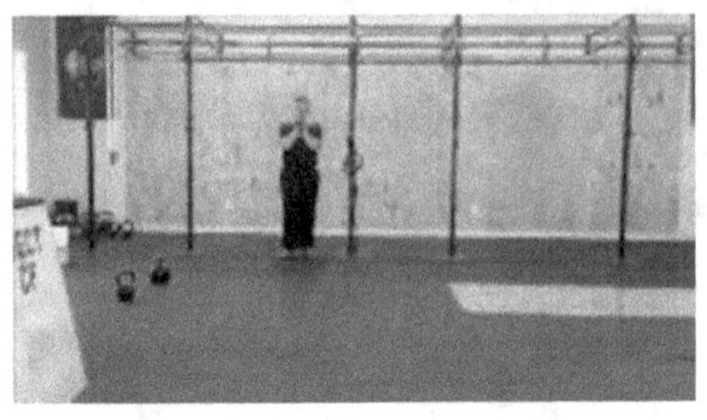 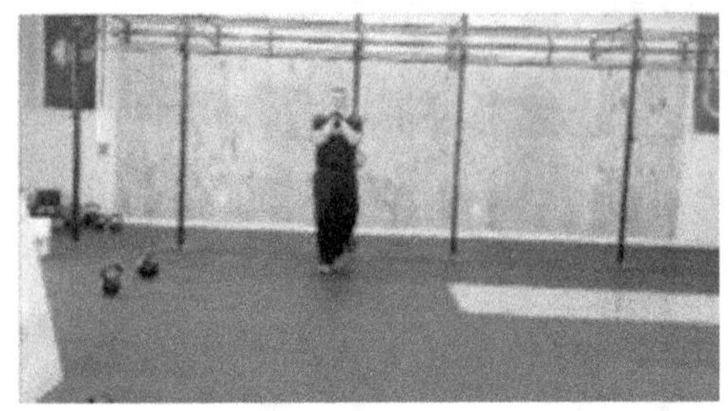

Movement :

1. Start with the bells in the gathered position.
2. Make sure the handles are above your collarbones.
3. Keep the kettlebells close to your biceps.
4. Do not let the bells sag or bend.
5. Start walking.

Precautions : Make sure your path is free of obstacles and select a weight that you can move with safely.

Goblet Squat

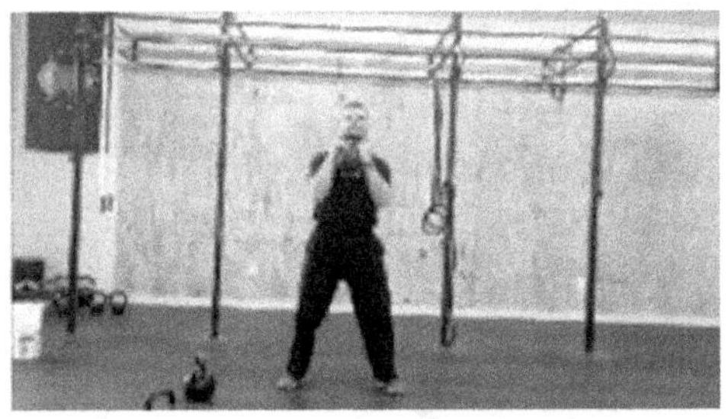 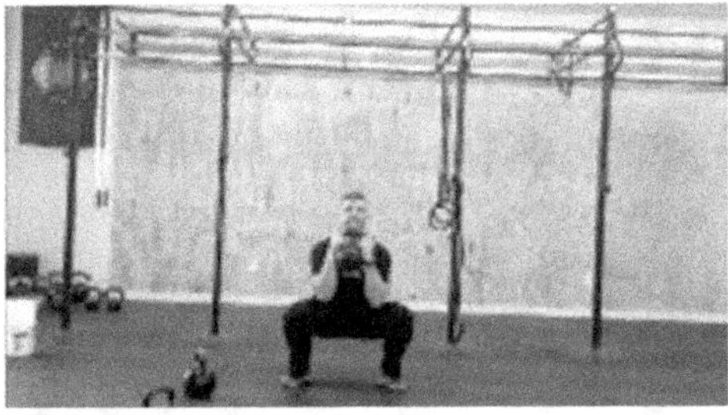

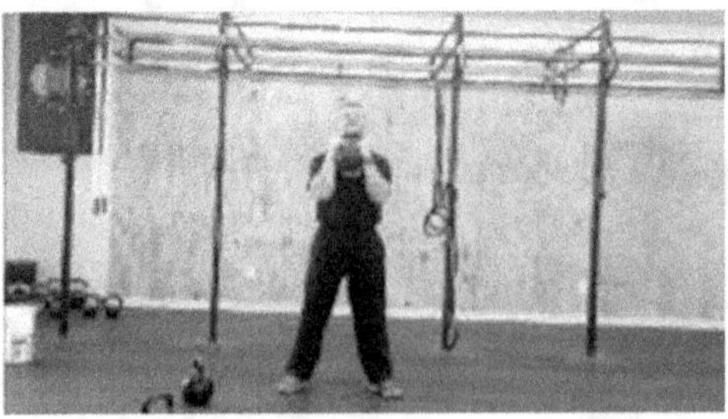

Movement :

1. Grab the bell by the horns.
2. Feet shoulder-width apart or slightly wider than shoulder-width apart.
3. Get down.
4. Keep your chest up while keeping your back as straight as possible.
5. Elbows tuck into knees with weight on heels not toes. 6. Stand up straight.

Precautions : Do not round your back and select an appropriate weight for your abilities.

Single Arm Deadlift

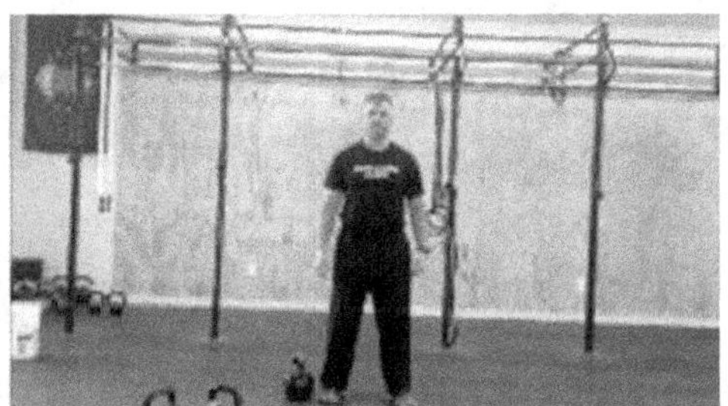
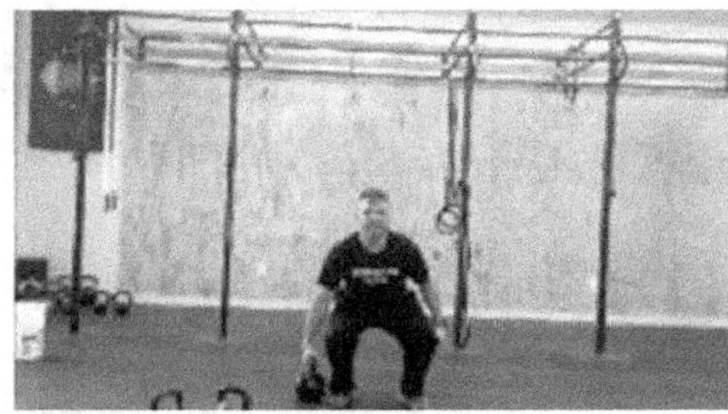

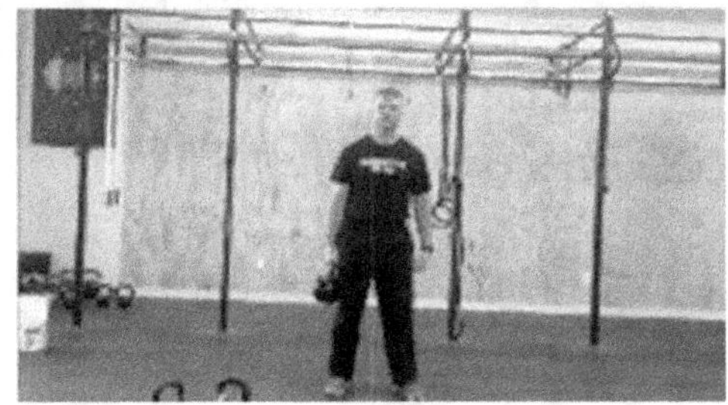

Movement :

1. Performed like a deadlift but with the weight by your side.
2. Bell will also be with your ankle.
3. Bend your waist and knees while keeping your back straight.
4. Stand straight without compensating on the non-weighted side.
5. Stand up straight.

Precautions : Your back should be straight and not rounded. Select a weight that is within your ability to lift safely.

Farmers Walk

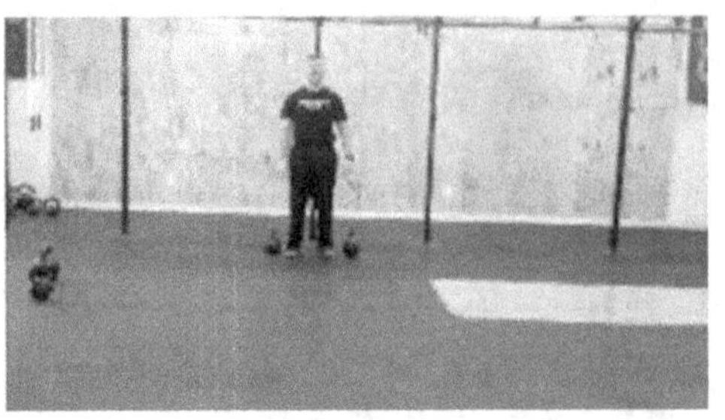
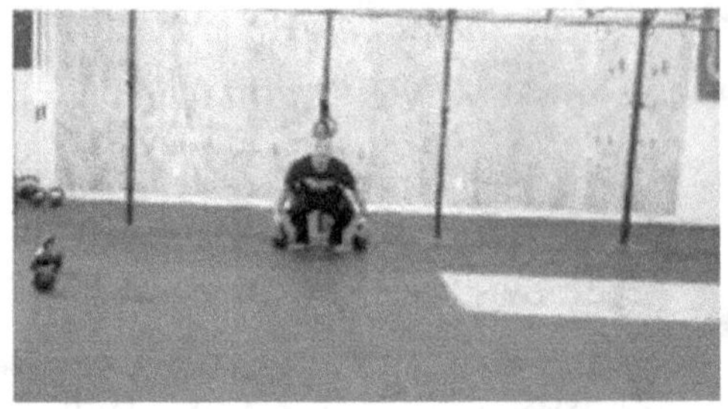

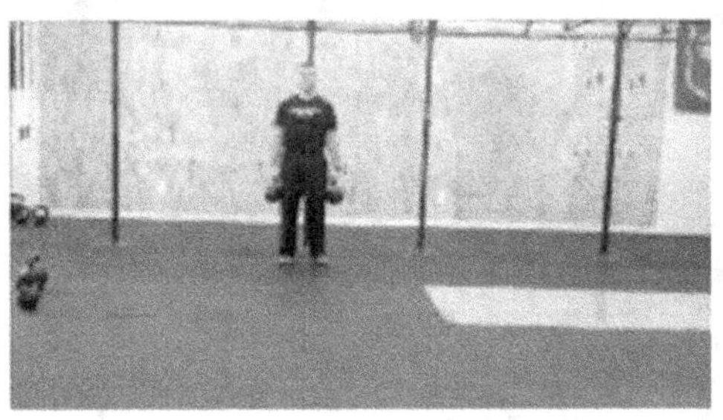

Movement :

1. Performed like a standard deadlift but with 2 bells at your side.
2. Use heavier weights so that the movement is challenging.
3. Start walking for the prescribed time.

Precautions : Do not round your back and always select a weight that you can move safely.

Swing Hand to Hand

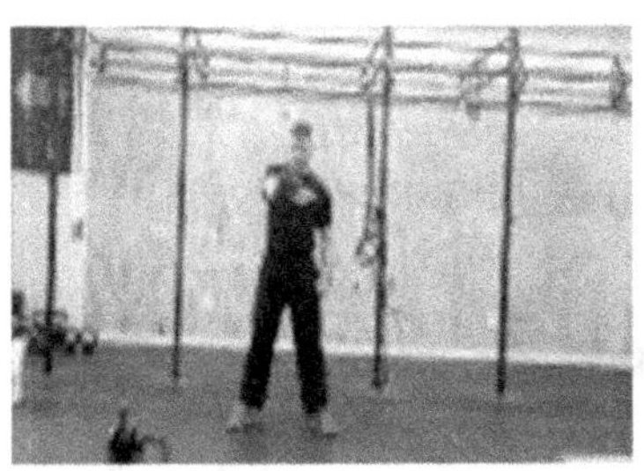
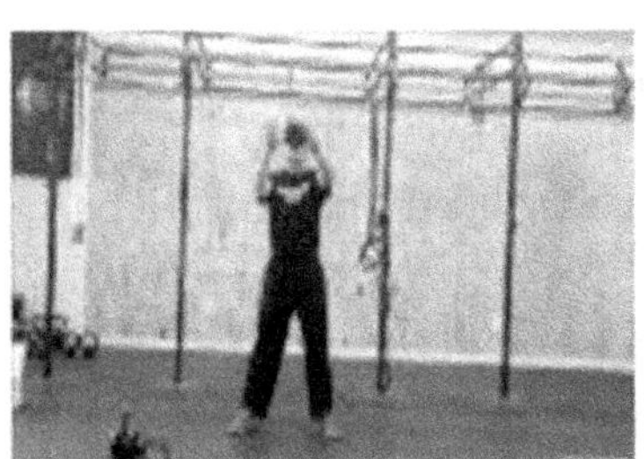

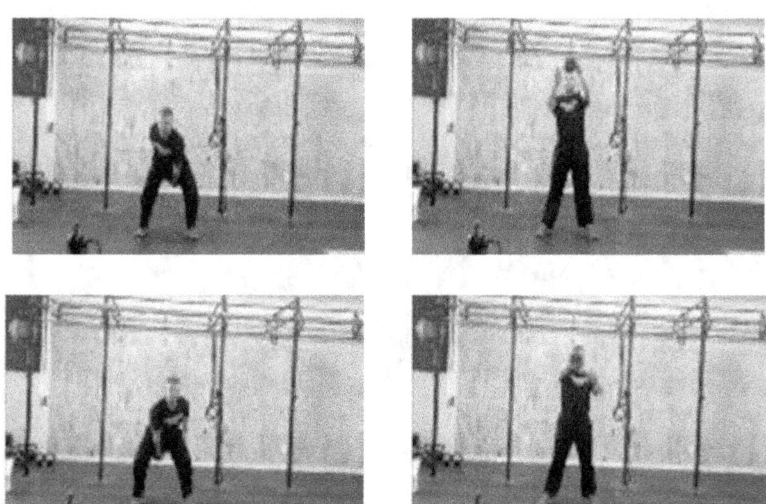

Movement :

Start with a regular swing, except now you will release the bell at the top of the swing.

Grab the bell with your other hand.

Move with purpose.

Precautions : If the bell is too far forward when you reach for it, let go and reset. Choose a weight that you can move safely.

Snatch Hand to Hand

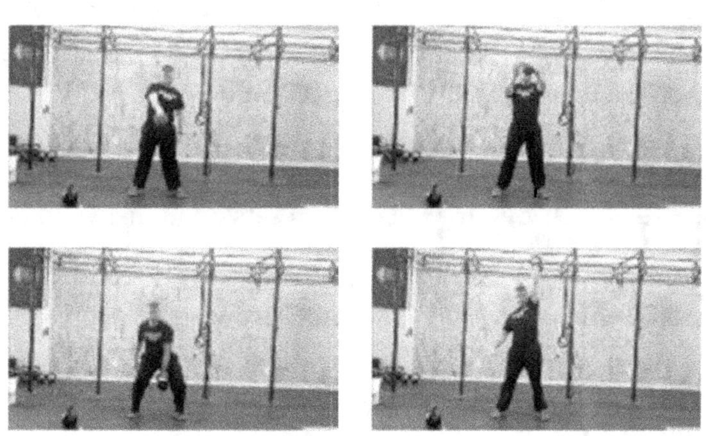

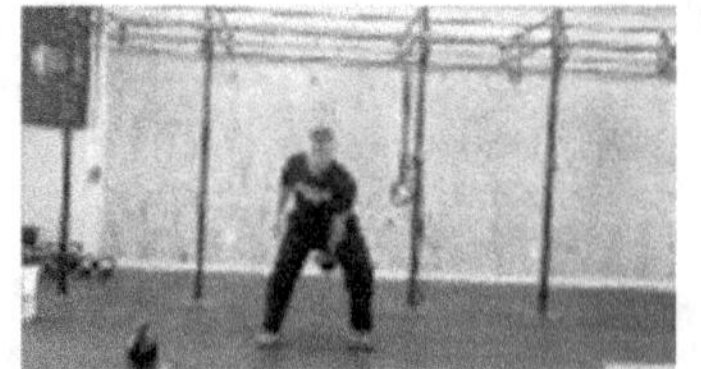
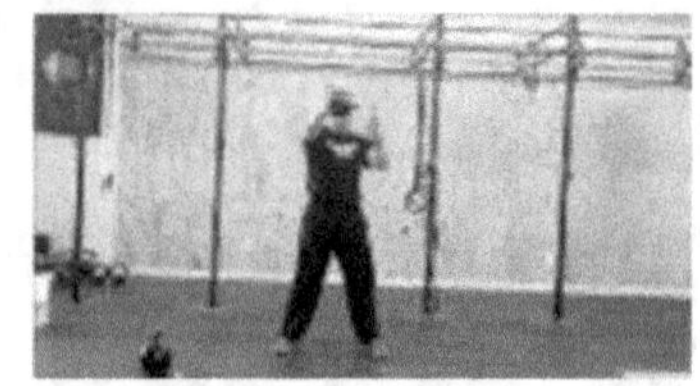

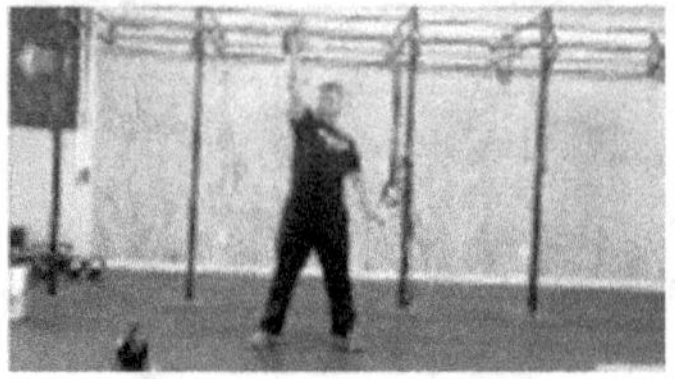

Movement :

1. Initiate the movement by performing the snatch with a swing.
2. Lower the bell with the same hand.
3. Lift the bell and receive the bell with your other hand.
4. Bring the bell back down and begin the transition as required.

Precautions : Make sure you don't round your back and select a weight that you can move safely.

Training history

Month 1

Day 1

- TGU-3 for alternate side

Overhead walk: 30 seconds each side

KB deadlift 4x5 choose weight , focus on hinge and lockout Swing scales- 3 bells of different sizes, 8 reps each x4 Carrying case - 3 sets of: 30 heavier bells

Single Arm Deadlifts 4x5 per arm Single Arm Swings - 4x8 per side

5x Board: 30

Detailed explanation:

TGU-3 ea. Alternate side. Here you want to focus on hitting each position in the movement. Do the left side then the right side until you do a total of 6 TGU. Work with a weight that you can handle safely. This is not a move that is done quickly, but rather an intentional movement. There is nothing wrong with using even something as light as your sneaker for the first 2 weeks, to learn the movement.

O/H KB Walk 30 seconds each side. Choose your weight carefully here . You will be moving with the weight above your head for a total of 30 seconds. Make sure to lock out that arm that is above your head. Walk normally.

- **Kettlebell raises 4 x 5.**

Choose an appropriate weight, focus on the hinge and the block. When it says 4 x 5 you will do 4 sets of 5. There is no predetermined rest period here. If you choose a weight that is neither too light nor too heavy, you will most likely only need to rest 1 minute.

- **Swing Ladders** - 3 bells of different sizes, 8 reps x 4.

If you are just starting out with kettlebells, start light. For men a 35 bell is probably the best and for women a 25 bell. Start with the lightest weight and do 8 two-handed swings, then move up to the medium weight and do 8 two-handed swings, then move up to the heaviest weight and do 8 two-handed swings. You will rest and do this again 3 more times.

- **Carry in your suitcase** : 3 sets of 30 seconds.

I would use my non-dominant hand first, then dominant, then non-dominant. If you need to rest, just lower the weight, rest, and go again.

- Single Arm **Deadlift 4 x 5 per arm.**

Focus on not compensating with the arm that is not lifting the weight. Make sure your back is straight. Do 5 reps on one arm, then 5 reps on the other arm. Rest the required amount and repeat 3 more times. Choose a challenging weight here .

- Single arm **swings 4 x 8 per side.**

Start with any arm, 8 with one arm, 8 with the other arm, rest if needed, repeat 3 more times. Make sure you select a weight you can safely move.

- **Plank** 5 x: 30 seconds. Chances are you won't be able to hold the plank for 30 seconds. That's okay, if you can only do 10 seconds, rest do 10

Day 2

TGU-hold each position for 5 seconds, 2 on each side

2 hand swings 5x10 Hip flexor stretch

hand swing 8L and 8R 6 goblet squats

Repeat 1 hand swing and glasses x4

- **Hand to hand swings**

Do 20 swings, go into: 30 plank reps x4

Farmers walk 4 sets of: 30 to: 45 seconds

Detailed explanation:

Turkish Get-Up Pause in ea. Position 5 seconds, 2 ea. Side.Here

you will stop on your forearm, palm, knee, and feet, and do the same on the way down. Focus on really feeling each position. Make sure to select a light weight. There is nothing wrong with using even something as light as your sneaker for the first 2 weeks, to learn the movement.

swings 5 x 10. You will do 10 reps with a weight you can safely handle. Rest for a short time, then do it 4 more times.

Hip flexor stretch. Really take the time to stretch each side. Focus on your entire body here.

- **Hand Swing 8L & 8R/6 Goblet Squats** .

You will do 8 swings with your left hand, then 8 with your right hand, and with the same weight you will move to the right performing 6 goblet squats. Rest for less than a minute and repeat 3 more times.

Do 20 hand-over-hand swings, then 30 seconds in the plank. Make sure you have practiced this move before doing it for the first time. If you are doing it at home, make sure there is nothing that can be broken. If you miss the bell, let it go and start over. After you have completed 20 body-to-body swings, you will immediately do 30 seconds in the plank and immediately begin the 20 body-to-body swings. You will do this for a total of 4 rounds.

- **Farmers Walk** -4 sets of 30 seconds to 45 seconds.

Choose a weight that is heavy enough to be challenging, but not so heavy that you have to put it down after 15 seconds. After hitting 30 to 45 seconds, lower the weight, recover, and repeat 3 more times.

Day 3

TGU standing, walk for: 30 seconds then go down, repeat on the way down

KB break - 4x5

KB oscillates 30/30 for 10 minutes

Goblet squat 6 reps, at the end of the 6th rep curl the kb 6 times for the horns, repeat 4 times

- **Swings** 30/30 1 arm.

Swing and then rest for: 30, repeat for 8 minutes

- **Hip flexor stretch**

Detailed explanation:

Turkish Get-Up Standing position Walk for 30 seconds then step down, repeat for the other arm. Do a Turkish get-up, then walk for 30 seconds, stop, step down, switch arms and repeat.

Kettlebell Deadlift 4 x 5. Do 5 reps with a weight that is not light, but not too heavy that you can't complete 4 sets. After doing 5 reps, rest for about 1 minute, then do 3 more reps . Make sure your back is straight, inhale on the way down, and exhale on the way up.

- **Kettlebell** swings 30/30 for 10 minutes.

You will do 30 seconds of 2 arm swings , rest for 30 seconds, and do this for a total of 10 minutes.

- **Goblet Squat 6 Reps** , grab the kettlebell by the horns 6x.

Repeat 4 times. Then you will do 6 goblet squats, sit into the squat, then do 6 bicep curls with the bell. Do this 3 more times. Don't be too aggressive with the weight here. Select a weight you can curl with versus a weight you can goblet squat with.

- Hip flexor **stretch .**

Really focus on a solid full body stretch here. Try to build up 20 seconds per side. I love this stretch!

Day 4

TGU, alternate each side for a total of 10 minutes

10 2 hand swings 8R and 8L 1 arm swing 10 goblet squats

20 hand-to-hand swings: 30 overhead walk L/R: 30 suitcase carry L/R

Repeat 4-6 times above for the time

Detailed explanation:

Turkish Get-Up, Alt ea. Side for a total of 10 minutes. Be careful with your weight selection here as you will be constantly moving from arm to arm and up. Don't focus on speed. Feel each step to get this movement right.

10 Two Handed Swings 8R & 8L 1 Arm Swing 10 Goblet

- Squats

20 hand-to-hand swings 30 seconds of overhead walking L/R 30 seconds of carrying suitcase L/R Repeat 4-6 times at a time

The goal on this day is to move from one exercise to the next without resting. Once you complete the round, rest, recharge, and set a goal to complete 4 to 6 rounds.

Month 2
Day 1

TGU-use a heavier bell if possible 6 total, 3 on each side alternating

1 swing, 1 snatch in the overhead walk for :15 2 swings, 2 snatches in the overhead walk for :15

3 swings, 3 snatches in the overhead walk for :15 4 swings, 4 snatches in the overhead walk for :15

Repeat above x5

Goblet squat- pause at the bottom position for :5 then come back up. 5x5

Kb rack walks

5 sets of :30

Detailed explanation:

- Get up Turkish Use a heavier bell if possible.

Do a total of 6, 3 on each side alternating. Now that you have been following the program for a month, you should be able to do more weight. Obviously, select a weight that is safe for your abilities. 1 swing, 1 jerk overhead walk for 15 seconds 2 swings, 2 jerks overhead walk for 15 seconds 3 swings, 3 jerks 4 overhead walk for 15 seconds swing, 4 jerks overhead walk for 15 seconds Repeat above for a total of 5 times

Here's how the workout works: You'll swing, snatch, walk for 15 seconds, then do 4 swings/snatches, then rest if needed and do it 4 more times. Keep the rest period as short as possible. Really push yourself here.

Goblet Squat-Pause in the Bottom position for 5 seconds, then come up 5 x 5. Here you will do 1 goblet squat, sit in the bottom position for 5 seconds, come up and do this 5 times. Rest if necessary, then repeat 4 more times.

Kettlebell Rack Walks 5 sets of 30 seconds :Rack the weight, and

walk for 30 seconds. Keep the rest short, then do 4 more times.

Day 2

TGU 8 minutes total, alternating each side

Clean and press 5x5

Double kb front squat 5x5

Push-up 4 sets of perfect shape

20 swings, 20 hand-to-hand swings , : 30 racket walk. repeat x4

Detailed explanation:

- Turkish Get-Up 8 minutes total, alternating each side.

reminder here, Just don't focus on speed, focus on movement during the Get-up. A slightly heavier weight than you can safely handle will cause your core to have extra work!

- Clean and press 5 x 5.

Do a Clean, then press it and do it for 5 reps, rest, then do 4 more. You will be able to clean much more than you can press. Base your press weight here on this movement .

- Double Kettlebell Front Squat 5 x 5.

Make sure you load the weight, keep your back straight, do 5 reps rest and 4 more times. Choose your weight wisely.

- Push-up 4 sets of perfect shape.

This is really a test of your mental toughness. Do as many pushups as you can with perfect form, rest, and repeat 3 more times. Record the number of pushups, so in the next 3 weeks you will know if you are progressing. Focus on form here NOT speed. Really push here.

20 swings, 20 hand-to-hand swings, 30 seconds of rack walking ,

repeat 4x.You should try to use the same weight for this. Then do 20 two-handed swings, then 20 hand-over-hand swings and finally walk the rack for 30 seconds, rest if needed and repeat 3 more times. Try to keep the rest period short .

Day 3

Overhead walk 4x :30 for each arm. Suitcase carries 4x :30 for each arm

10 1 arm swing L/R 10 snatch L/R

20 hand to hand snatches

repeat x4

2 handballs, 8 minutes total 40/20

Detailed explanation:

Overhead Walk 4 x 30 seconds per arm

Suitcase Carry 4 x 30 seconds per arm 10 1 Arm swing left then right 10 Snatch left then right

20 Snatch hand to hand Repeat 4x

Move from one exercise to the next without resting. You should know how to do hand-to-hand snatches before attempting this. After a round, rest for a short time, catch your breath, and repeat 3 more times. Really push yourself here!

Then: 2 Hand Swings @ 40/20, 8 minutes total. A real test here, do 40 seconds of 2 hand swings, rest 20 seconds and do a total of 8 times.

Day 4

1 TGU per arm

20 2- hand swings 10 R and 10 L 1 one-arm swing 8 goblet squats Snatches 8 L and 8 R

2 TGU per arm

rack :30

Repeat 4-6 times at a time .

Detailed explanation:

1 Turkish Get-Up per arm. Challenge yourself here! 20 2- Hand Swings

10 right arm swings and 10 left arm swings

1 8 goblet squats

8 left snatches and 8 right 2 Turkish get-ups Each arm walks for 30 seconds Repeat 4-6 times at a time .

Notes: Get-ups should not be rushed. Feel each position. Move from one exercise to the next with a challenging weight, rest, and aim for 4-6 sets.

If you have completed 8 weeks of the training program, you can always start over from week 1 and do another 8 weeks. You can add more weight, shorten the rest periods. I will be developing more intense kettlebell workouts in the future.

Chapter 5: Living a Healthy Lifestyle

Reaching your goal weight is a big accomplishment, but sticking to it is crucial to not lose your progress! Planning ahead is key to avoid ruining all your hard work. Celebrating your success will be even more rewarding if you are able to maintain your new healthy and active lifestyle.

Never skip meals!

Skipping meals can be a big mistake. Your body, sensing the lack of food, may activate conservation mechanisms and store fat as a reserve. To avoid this, continue to follow a regular eating routine, as you have done up until now. If you skip a meal, you are very likely to end up bingeing at the next one, compromising portion control and hunger.

Keep variety in your diet

A balanced and varicd diet is essential to provide your body with all the nutrients it needs. Be sure to include foods like whole grains, fruits, vegetables, and lean proteins . This approach will not only keep you healthy, but it will help you feel energetic and protect your immune system. Additionally, a diet rich in fiber, vitamins, and minerals will help support your metabolism and fat loss.

Constant and dynamic training

Don't stop training! One of the most common mistakes is to abandon exercise once you've reached your goals. Remember that your body needs constant stimulation to avoid stagnation. Change up your routine every now and then: add kettlebell training sessions, resistance exercises and cardiovascular workouts.

These are especially effective for burning fat, improving muscle tone, and strengthening the cardiovascular system. Kettlebell training, in particular, offers a full-body workout that increases strength and speeds up your metabolism, helping you continue to burn fat even after your workout.

Manage your calorie intake

Once you reach your ideal weight, it's natural to wonder how to adjust your calorie intake. Increase it gradually, not abruptly . Start by adding 250 calories per day and monitor your weight weekly. If you continue to lose weight, add another 250 calories until you find your balance. Conversely, if you start to gain weight, reduce your calorie intake by 100 calories at a time until your weight stabilizes. This approach will allow you to maintain your new weight in a healthy and sustainable way.

Constant hydration

Don't forget to drink water! Maintaining proper hydration is essential for the proper functioning of the body. Water not only aids digestion, but it helps maintain high energy levels, removes toxins and supports weight loss. Aim to drink at least 8 glasses of water a day, especially if you exercise regularly.

Frequent and balanced meals

Continuing to eat five or six small meals a day is a healthy habit you should maintain. This method keeps your metabolism active and helps you avoid binge eating. Eating smaller portions more often helps you manage hunger better and keeps your energy levels stable. Make sure to keep portions under control to avoid falling back into old habits.

Avoid junk food

Now that you have developed healthy eating habits, avoid falling back into junk food consumption. You have discovered how healthy and nutritious foods can satisfy your cravings. Continue to include fruits and vegetables in your diet, aiming for 6-8 servings per day. These foods are rich in antioxidants, vitamins and fiber that support your health and help you maintain a healthy weight.

Don't forget your vitamins

Supplementing your diet with daily vitamins and minerals is essential to ensure you are getting all the nutrients your body needs. Vitamins not only support your immune system, but they also play a key role in weight maintenance and disease prevention.

In short, maintaining your new weight requires discipline, but with the right strategies, you can live a healthy and happy lifestyle in the long run. Implement these tips into your daily routine and stay motivated to continue your journey to a healthier, fitter body, making health a long-term priority. With effective workouts like the kettlebell workout and a balanced diet, you will not only feel and look your best, but you will ensure a healthy, fit future.

The secrets to a healthy and well life

Everyone wants to live a long, healthy, and fit life, avoiding serious illnesses and enjoying a general state of well-being. While we cannot predict every eventuality, there are many strategies we can adopt to improve the quality of our lives and prevent many health problems.

Prevention and early diagnosis

Prevention is one of the keys to living a longer, healthier life. Many people tend to neglect routine medical visits, such as annual checkups with their primary care physician or regular visits to the dentist. These regular checkups, however, are crucial for identifying potential health problems at an early stage, allowing for timely intervention . Don't wait until pain or symptoms become unbearable; make prevention a priority.

Family history and health monitoring

Knowing your family history can make a difference in managing your health. If you have a family history of diseases such as diabetes, cancer, or heart disease, it is essential to tell your doctor so that they can monitor you on a targeted and regular basis. Specific tests and frequent check-ups can help you spot warning signs early.

Positive Relationships and Mental Health

Mental well-being is closely linked to physical health. The relationships we cultivate with our partners, family and friends are essential to our psychological balance. Dedicate time to healthy relationships, reducing the risk of isolation and depression. The positive emotions stimulated by these interactions can also help reduce the level of cortisol, the stress hormone, improving your immune system.

Sleep and recovery

Sleep at least 7-9 hours a night. Sleep is the best regenerator for your body and mind. Adequate rest is essential to maintain high energy levels, improve concentration, and promote muscle recovery. In addition, chronic sleep deprivation can increase the risk of chronic diseases such as type 2 diabetes and hypertension. Take the importance of sleep seriously for a long and healthy life.

Stress Management

Stress is a part of everyday life, but how you manage it makes a difference. High levels of unmanaged stress can lead to health problems such as high blood pressure, heart disease, and a compromised immune system. Practices such as meditation, yoga , and walking outdoors can help reduce the impact of stress. It is also important to avoid overloading yourself by maintaining a healthy balance between work, family, and leisure time.

Work-life balance

Maintaining a work-life balance is essential to well-being. Don't get so caught up in your work commitments that you neglect your family, hobbies, and passions . Cultivating personal interests and spending time with loved ones can dramatically improve your quality of life, reducing stress and promoting happiness.

Benefits of a Healthy Lifestyle

The benefits of maintaining a healthy lifestyle go beyond physical appearance. Being fit and healthy allows you to have more energy, improve emotional and mental well-being, and reduce the risk of chronic diseases. Eating a balanced diet, getting regular exercise, and managing stress positively can transform your health.

Physical health

Maintaining a healthy body allows you to better face the challenges of everyday life. Good physical fitness helps you move better, reducing the risk of injury and disease. In addition, an active lifestyle reduces the risk of developing diseases such as obesity, heart disease and diabetes. Include the use of kettlebells in your routine, a versatile and effective workout to burn fat and improve muscle strength.

Mental health and the importance of psychological well-being

Mental health is equally crucial. Managing emotions and stress effectively is essential to avoiding physical health problems such as high blood pressure and heart disease. Find activities that help you relax and improve your mental health, such as meditating, listening to relaxing music, or practicing breathing exercises.

Disease prevention through nutrition

Diet plays a major role in disease prevention. Eating a diet rich in fruits, vegetables, whole grains, and lean proteins can reduce the risk of chronic disease. Include foods like avocados, salmon, berries, and green leafy vegetables, which are rich in antioxidants and nutrients essential for cardiovascular health and the prevention of diseases like cancer and diabetes.

regular exercise

Exercise is an essential part of a healthy lifestyle. Regular workouts, like kettlebells, can accelerate fat loss, improve muscle mass, and increase endurance. Kettlebells are a versatile tool that provide a full-body workout, burning calories and improving cardiovascular health. Supplement your workout with a balanced aerobic and strength training routine for optimal results.

Live long and healthy

Adopting a healthy lifestyle can help you live longer and with a higher quality of life. Daily choices, such as nutrition, physical activity, and stress management, significantly impact the prevention of chronic diseases and the maintenance of a healthy and vital body. It's never too late to start taking care of yourself.

Chapter 6:
Best Dietary Supplements: What to Look for and How to Choose

If you want to transform your body or are looking for the **best fat burners** and **cutting edge anti-aging supplements** , it is essential to find a company you can trust. Quality is key, and investing in products that deliver on their promises is the key to maximizing your kettlebell training results.

Many of us have had disappointing experiences in vitamin stores, being pushed to buy supplements that have brought no real benefit. This is because, unfortunately, the quality of food is decreasing. The use of quality supplements, especially those aimed at improving **body composition** and **metabolic health** , becomes crucial to ensuring vitality and longevity.

Why Supplements Are Essential

Today more than ever, integrating your daily diet is essential. We can no longer rely on food alone to get all the nutrients we need. Daily vitamin supplements can really make a difference in your appearance and overall well-being. **Fat burning vitamins** and **metabolic support supplements** are powerful tools that speed up the fat loss process, improve energy, and support vital body functions.

If you're looking to **burn fat** and improve muscle definition with kettlebells, consider adding a high-quality supplement to maximize your results. **Fat loss supplements** like those containing **CLA (conjugated linoleic acid)** , **caffeine** , or **green tea extract** can boost your metabolism and promote **thermogenesis** , or the process of burning calories.

The Right Supplements for Men and Women

Whether you are a man or a woman , there are specific supplements that can support your well-being. It is essential to choose natural supplements that are easily absorbed by the body and not synthetic ones, avoiding those that pass through the system without providing real benefits.

Essential Supplements for Women

Women , in particular, have unique nutritional needs that **are** often not met through daily nutrition. **Vitamin and mineral supplements specifically for** women can help balance hormones, improve energy, and support mood. A suitable vitamin should help maintain hormonal balance, support energy levels, and improve the quality of daily life, especially during times of stress or hormonal changes.

If you are unable to consume at least 10 servings of fruits and vegetables a day, it is highly recommended to supplement. Vitamins such as vitamin **D** , **Magnesium** and **omega-3s** are essential for women's health. These supplements, in addition to maintaining stable energy levels, help protect bones and prevent deficiencies that can lead to health problems as we age.

Supplements For Fat Loss And Wellness

Fat loss vitamins and supplements need to be chosen carefully. It is important to select supplements that promote **lipolysis** , or the breakdown of fat, and improve **insulin sensitivity** . Products such as **carnitine** and **Raspberry ketones** are known for their fat burning effect and support fat oxidation during exercise.

Furthermore, natural supplements such as **Green tea** and **guarana** can improve fat burning during kettlebell training sessions, promoting greater endurance and speeding up muscle recovery.

The New Generation of Supplements: Natural and Non-Synthetic

With the increase in daily stress, it is essential to find supplements that not only help you burn fat, but also maintain emotional balance . The new generation of supplements are formulated to be easily digestible, avoiding common side effects such as stomach upset that often accompany synthetic supplements. Today, you can find products that provide all the essential nutrients without overloading your body with artificial additives.

In addition, **women -specific vitamin supplementation** must also take into account the nutrients lost during physical activity. Supplements containing **vitamin C , biotin** , and **zinc** not only help improve skin and hair, but also support the immune system and promote muscle tissue regeneration.

If you want to get the most out of your kettlebell workouts and reach your fat loss goals, you can't ignore the importance of nutritional supplements. Choosing natural **fat burners that are formulated specifically for** your body can make the difference between mediocre results and noticeable success.

For Men Only: Keep Your Confidence at Its Best!

Men also face unique challenges that need to be carefully managed. Among these, a daily vitamin supplement can make all the difference in ensuring that the body receives all the nutrients it needs. With the presence of testosterone, men face specific issues such as prostate and urinary health, which can develop into serious health problems if not addressed early.

Maintaining an attractive and confident appearance is crucial for a man, as self-esteem is closely tied to his social perception. It is well known that men receive less "social proof" than women, which makes it even more important to always present yourself at your best to maintain high levels of confidence. Daily vitamin supplements that offer essential ingredients to boost your metabolism, burn fat faster, and get you in shape are very rare among the standard multivitamins available on the market.

Ensuring adequate intake of essential fatty acids, vitamins, enzymes and amino acids can be difficult, especially when you struggle to consume the right amount of food throughout the day to meet your body's needs.

Liquid diets for weight loss? Why not choose a Meal Replacement?

If you're struggling to lose fat, relying on a liquid diet is not advisable. In fact, many people don't eat enough, mistakenly believing that drastically cutting calories will lead to weight loss. This is only partly true. Eating less can work for a period of 10 to 14 days, after which the body adapts, slowing down the metabolism to conserve energy. This mechanism, known as homeostasis, can lead to the so-called "yo-yo syndrome" of dieting, characterized by a rapid regain of lost weight.

Repeating this pattern can damage your metabolism, further pushing your weight loss goals further away. Many people choose liquid diets to lose weight, but this is not an optimal solution. Why? The reason is simple: balance is essential to achieving a lean and fit body. Instead of a "liquid diet," opt for a healthy meal replacement. Why is this so important? Because speeding up your metabolism means consuming enough food to keep your body constantly active, burning calories even while digestion is taking place.

Going on a liquid diet for every meal could turn your body into a calorie-burning machine, but at what cost? No one wants to live on drinks alone. Eating solid, nutritious meals is key. Real food provides essential nutrients and a satisfaction that liquids simply can't provide.

Which meal replacement should you choose?

When choosing a meal replacement, make sure it tastes good. A bad-tasting formula could reduce your motivation to stick with it. Personally, I prefer something that is not only nutritious, but also tasty. Here are some essentials that a good meal replacement should contain:

- **Protein** : Between 30 and 40 grams per serving. Adequate protein intake is crucial for muscle recovery and maintaining an active metabolism. Avoid excessive amounts, as the body can only absorb up to 40 grams of protein per meal.
- **No artificial sweeteners** : Many products contain ingredients like aspartame, which can cause side effects like headaches. Opt for a meal replacement that is free of artificial sweeteners to maintain overall well-being.
- **Low Fat** : You don't want to take in excess fat, especially if your goal is to burn it.

A good meal replacement will provide you with all the essential nutrients without compromising your progress. That's why it's essential to always read labels carefully and consult a nutritionist.

Natural Testosterone Supplements

As men age, their testosterone levels decline. This hormone is essential for maintaining muscle mass, reducing body fat, and supporting sex drive and energy. Over the past few decades, the fitness world has been looking for natural ways to boost testosterone, and now these supplements are finally available to the general public.

Increasing your testosterone levels can bring many benefits: increased self-confidence , a more sculpted body, improved physical and sexual performance. However, using testosterone injections without a prescription is not only illegal, but can cause serious side effects such as testicular atrophy and hormonal imbalances.

There are natural solutions, such as herbs and supplements based on safe ingredients, that stimulate testosterone production in a balanced way and without side effects. This is why it is important to look for natural and certified products to improve health without risks.

To achieve real results in your physical transformation, it is essential to follow a balanced eating plan that includes real, nutritious food, quality supplements, and effective workouts . Avoid extreme diets and focus on on adopting healthy and sustainable habits in the long term. Your fitness and health will improve as a result, leading you to the body and confidence you desire.

The Holistic Solution for a Fit Body: Burn Fat with Kettlebells

If you're interested in holistic health, you know that the traditional approach to weight loss may not always be the best option. There are more natural and effective ways to boost testosterone production and improve metabolism, without the harmful and potentially dangerous side effects. Kettlebells offer a great solution for those who want to lose fat, gain strength, and improve their overall well-being.

In fact, many men, despite having lower testosterone levels as they age, do not have access to hormone therapy. It is therefore essential to consider natural solutions that can help keep the metabolism active and promote healthy fat loss, such as kettlebell training.

Testosterone's Crucial Role in Metabolism: Why Fat Accumulates and How to Fight It

Testosterone plays a central role in managing body fat and metabolism. As men age, testosterone levels tend to decline, which leads to a slower metabolism. This can result in unwanted fat accumulation, especially in the abdominal area. Men with low testosterone often struggle with weight gain and a reduced ability to burn calories.

This is where kettlebells come in. Kettlebell workouts, which combine strength and cardio, can boost your metabolism and promote effective fat burning. Naturally increasing testosterone levels through targeted training not only improves your metabolism, but also helps preserve lean muscle mass, which is essential for maintaining a healthy, lean body.

Revolutionize Your Workout: The Power of Kettlebells to Burn Fat and Tone Your Body

If you have tried conventional diets or exercises without success, kettlebells may be the solution you are looking for. Thanks to their versatility, they can be used for a complete workout that involves all the major muscle groups, while increasing endurance and strength.

Kettlebell workouts stimulate the natural release of testosterone, which promotes fat loss and improves muscle definition. Using natural supplements to support hormone levels can increase energy, improve mood, and promote a winning mentality. A positive attitude is key when it comes to reaching your fitness goals, and testosterone plays a key role in this.

It's never too late to take back control: your masculine energy at its peak

If you've noticed a decrease in energy, a reduction in stamina, or a loss of confidence, it's time to restore your testosterone levels. Kettlebell training, combined with natural supplements, can help you regain your lost vitality and enjoy a life full of energy and vigor again. Don't underestimate the importance of feeling at your best.

Kettlebell Trainers

Athletes and fitness enthusiasts know how essential it is to provide the body with the right nutrients. When you train intensely, such as with kettlebells, your body needs an optimal amount of vitamins, minerals, and other nutrients to maintain peak performance and burn fat efficiently.

Often, the so-called "wall" that many athletes encounter in their journey is due to a lack of nutrients. Supplementing your diet with the best supplements for athletes can make the difference between stagnant progress and continuous improvement. Kettlebells , with their intense energy consumption, require adequate nutritional support to maximize results.

Overcoming the "Wall" with the Right Nutrition and Training Strategies

Throughout my fitness career, I have often found myself stuck, unable to see any progress despite my best efforts. What has made the difference is a combination of high-quality nutritional supplementation and kettlebell training aimed at fat loss. Instead of wasting time on ineffective diets, I have found that a well-structured routine and adequate supplementation are the key to achieving tangible results.

Nutritional supplements for athletes not only support muscle growth, but also provide the energy needed to tackle intense training sessions. When you choose to supplement your daily diet with quality products, you can achieve a faster and longer-lasting physical transformation.

The Science Behind Kettlebell Fat Burning: How to Maintain a Lean, Ripped Body

Kettlebells offer a scientifically backed approach to burning fat and building lean muscle. As you gain muscle mass, your metabolism speeds up, allowing your body to burn more calories even at rest. This is the secret to staying lean and fit in the long run.

Due to their ability to engage multiple muscle groups at once, kettlebells are ideal for those looking to achieve fast and effective fat loss results. By incorporating kettlebell workouts into your fitness regimen, you can maximize fat loss, improve strength, and maintain an enviable physique.

Gluconeogenesis: A Metabolic Challenge to Face Post-Workout

If you're unfamiliar with the concept of the " 60- minute metabolic window," it's the period immediately following a workout when your body desperately needs to replenish nutrients, especially glycogen lost during exercise.

Glycogen is the body's main carbohydrate store, which is essential for energy during exercise. When you exercise intensely, your body depletes these stores, and after more than 20 minutes of exercise, it goes into "fat-burning" mode. After the activity, however, your body goes into a recovery phase, requiring glycogen to restore its optimal function.

The Danger of Gluconeogenesis

If you don't replenish your carbs quickly after your workout, your body will activate a process called gluconeogenesis, where it creates carbs from unconventional sources, like muscle protein. This is the worst nightmare for anyone who wants to burn fat and preserve muscle mass: your body may use up your recently trained muscles to replenish glycogen. This is a mechanism that hinders your progress, negatively impacting both fat loss and muscle growth.

Not only does gluconeogenesis take away muscle mass—the primary stimulator of metabolism—it can also disrupt your long-term metabolic balance. A body that burns muscle for energy enters a vicious cycle that slows your progress toward weight loss and overall wellness.

Preventing Gluconeogenesis: The Importance of Post- Workout Supplements Nutritional supplements can play a key role in blocking gluconeogenesis, providing the body with the nutrients it needs for recovery. Specific supplements for athletes, combining carbohydrates and high-quality proteins, can prevent the body from using muscle tissue as an energy source.

Science at your service: discover solutions to optimize recovery Thanks to advances in sports nutrition, there are more and more solutions that allow you to recover faster, maintain muscle and accelerate fat loss. By choosing the right supplements, you can maximize the results of your kettlebell training, improving both your strength and your ability to burn fat. Discover how you can say goodbye to gluconeogenesis with the best supplements on the market.

The Role of Testosterone in Fat Loss for Men

For men, testosterone is a crucial ally in the fight against body fat. This hormone is essential not only for muscle mass and strength, but also for metabolism. Low testosterone levels can make it difficult to lose fat and maintain a lean physique.

Naturally increasing testosterone levels through a balanced diet and regular exercise can make a big difference. High-intensity workouts, such as kettlebells, are especially effective at boosting testosterone production. Three weekly workouts, combining strength and cardio, can boost your metabolism and improve your body composition.

Testosterone
Levels Eating a diet rich in lean protein, healthy fats, and complex carbohydrates is key. Avoid processed foods and refined sugars, which can lower testosterone levels.

Additionally, some supplements can support your efforts:

- Tribulus terrestris – An herb traditionally used to stimulate libido and increase testosterone levels.
- Zinc – Essential for testosterone production. Found in red meat, nuts, and seeds.
- Vitamin D – Low vitamin D levels are associated with reduced testosterone. Consider taking a supplement or getting some sun.

- D-Aspartic Acid (DAA) – An amino acid that aids in the synthesis of testosterone.
- Omega-3 – Improves insulin sensitivity and promotes testosterone production.
- Magnesium – A mineral that aids in the production of testosterone and is found in green leafy vegetables, nuts, and seeds.

Optimize recovery with a targeted routine

Kettlebell training, combined with targeted nutrition and the right supplement support , will allow you to burn fat faster and maintain healthy muscle mass. Remember to take supplements carefully and follow the recommended doses. Always consult a doctor or nutritionist before starting any supplement program .

With the right strategy, the combination of exercise and nutrition will help you maximize your efforts, boosting your metabolism and improving your body composition. If you are looking to improve your health and burn fat, increasing testosterone is a valuable weapon to exploit.

In conclusion, to achieve optimal fat loss results, it is essential to exercise regularly, eat a balanced diet, and adopt strategies to naturally boost testosterone. Approach gluconeogenesis with the right knowledge and products, and your body will emerge victorious, ready to reach its maximum physical potential.

Conclusion: Ready... set... go!

Now that you've learned how to transform your lifestyle and start losing weight effectively using kettlebells, it's time to take action. Everyone knows what to do: they read articles, follow programs, and realize that they have to put in the work to get results. But the truth is, even with all this information, the crucial step is often missing: action. Many people fail to get started on the path to a healthy lifestyle because their motivation wanes or they give in to unhealthy habits.

The key to success is consistency.

No program or exercise will ever be effective if there is no iron discipline and strong motivation to choose healthy foods and maintain a regular exercise regimen. Without real commitment, no amount of reading or affirmations like "Yes, I can do this!" will lead you to the desired change.

The first step is crucial.

It takes determination to get started and unwavering perseverance to stick with it. Many people get discouraged when results don't come right away. But here's the difference: Those who persevere , who continue to eat a balanced diet and practice kettlebell training will be able to achieve any goal, whether it's weight loss, increasing endurance, or improving performance in a specific sport.

Kettlebell training isn't just a fat burning method; it's a comprehensive approach to improving your functional strength, endurance, and mobility. Over time, you'll not only see physical improvements, but you'll also develop a stronger mindset and inner discipline. This confidence will translate into a positive attitude that will help you resist unhealthy temptations more easily and stay focused on your goals.

Start with small steps.

Don't try to do everything at once or lose 10 pounds in a week by riding a stationary bike. This will only lead to frustration and injury. Success is built gradually. You can start with simple brisk walks, then integrate kettlebell exercises to strengthen your body and prepare it for more challenging sessions in the weeks to come. This gradual approach will allow you to adapt physically and mentally, minimizing the risk of injury.

One of the most common mistakes people make when starting a workout program is doing too much, too soon. This can lead to intense muscle pain, injury, and eventually giving up on the plan altogether. It's crucial to listen to your body and find a pace that allows you to progress without overdoing it.

To avoid these pitfalls, it is advisable to establish a well-structured training program. If you feel unsure, you can consult a personal trainer who can help you create a personalized plan that suits your needs. Remember, simplicity is the key: there is no need to make the process complicated. If your main goal is weight loss, short sessions of kettlebell exercises combined with a healthy and controlled diet are sufficient.

Maintaining a positive attitude is essential.

Even when progress seems slow, keep working toward your goals. The results will come if you stay consistent and committed. As a new season approaches, this is the perfect time to make a concrete plan and take real steps toward a future of wellness and vitality. Don't forget that patience and consistency are the key ingredients for success.

Kettlebells: The Secret Weapon for Burning Fat and Toning Your Body .

These machines have become increasingly popular because they combine cardiovascular training with muscle strengthening, increasing metabolism and burning fat efficiently. They also improve posture, increase flexibility and strengthen stabilizing muscles, which are essential for preventing injuries.

Using kettlebells means you can train your entire body in relatively short, yet intense sessions, which is ideal for those who are short on time. Exercises like the swing or snatch engage a large number of muscle groups, making the workout extremely effective in terms of calorie burning. These dynamic movements will not only help you burn fat quickly, but will also improve your balance and functional strength.

Ready to get started?

Now you have all the knowledge you need to put a successful plan into action. Don't wait any longer. Get started today, set your goals, and take it one step at a time. With kettlebells as your primary tool, you'll be able to transform your body, improve your health, and feel your best.

Appendix : Revolutionary Kettlebell Activities - 2024 Edition

1. VR Kettlebell 360° Challenge

The VR Kettlebell 360 Challenge represents the pinnacle of technology and fitness fusion. This immersive experience uses virtual reality to transport users into breathtaking environments while they train with kettlebells.

- **How it works:**
    - Users wear a compatible VR headset and hold motion sensors on the kettlebells.
    - The VR app generates realistic scenarios, from the Grand Canyon to Martian landscapes.
    - Kettlebell exercises are integrated into the virtual environment, creating unique challenges (e.g., swinging kettlebells to "climb" a virtual mountain).
- **Benefits:**
    - Greater Engagement: The immersive environment distracts from fatigue, allowing for longer, more intense sessions.
    - Variety in training: Ever-changing scenarios and challenges prevent boredom.
    - Fitness Gamification: Game Elements Increase Motivation and Persistence.
- **Technology involved:**
    - 6- axis motion tracking .
    - Wireless kettlebell sensors that transmit data in real time.
    - AI-powered environment rendering software to create ever-changing scenarios.

2. Kettlebell Flow Choreography

Choreographic Kettlebell Flow is an innovative discipline that fuses the effectiveness of kettlebell training with the elegance and fluidity of dance.

- **Program structure:**

- live streaming sessions with certified instructors.
    - Progression from basic movements to complex sequences.
    - Integrating elements of yoga, pilates and martial arts for a holistic practice.
- **Dedicated App:**
    - Video tutorial library for every move.
    - Progress tracking system with AI motion analysis .
    - Social features to share achievements and challenge friends.
- **Benefits:**
    - Improved coordination and balance.
    - Development of functional strength and flexibility.
    - Increased calorie expenditure thanks to continuous movement.

3. Eco-Kettlebell Challenge

The Eco-Kettlebell Challenge combines fitness with respect for the environment, creating a positive impact on both your body and the planet.

- **Eco-Kettlebell Kit:**
    - Kettlebells made from recycled ocean plastic and biodegradable materials.
    - Ergonomic design to maximize comfort and performance.
    - Each kettlebell is unique, with a QR code that tells its "recycling story."
- **Environmental impact:**
    - Algorithm that converts calories burned into "green credits".
    - Collaboration with global reforestation organizations.
    - Personal dashboard showing cumulative environmental impact.
- **Training program:**
    - Thematic workouts based on environmental issues (e.g. "Ocean Clean-up HIIT").
    - Monthly challenges with eco-friendly prizes.
    - Integrated educational content on environmental issues.

4. Custom Genetic Kettlebell

The Kettlebell Genetic Custom program uses DNA analysis to create a training and nutrition plan tailored to each individual.

- **Process:**
    1. Sending the genetic analysis kit to your home.
    2. Sample analysis in state-of-the-art laboratories.
    3. Processing data with AI to create genetic fitness profile.
    4. Generate a personalized training and nutrition plan.
- **Elements of the plan:**
    - Recommendations on the type of kettlebell exercises best suited to your genetic profile.
    - Nutritional advice based on individual metabolic response.
    - Personalized recovery strategies.
- **Continuous updates:**
    - Quarterly recalibration of the plan based on progress.
    - Wearable data integration for more accurate analysis.
    - Virtual consultations with genetics and fitness experts.

5. Kettlebell AI Coach

Kettlebell AI Coach is a virtual personal trainer powered by advanced artificial intelligence, available 24/7.

- **Key Features:**
    - Real-time analysis of exercise form and execution.
    - Instant voice feedback for corrections and encouragement.
    - Dynamic program adaptation based on performance and recovery.
- **Technology:**
    - Using computer vision for motion analysis.
    - Machine learning algorithms to personalize recommendations.
    - Integration with smart home devices for an immersive experience.
- **Interaction:**
    - Conversational interface for questions and support.
    - Generate detailed post-workout reports.
    - Proactive tips to improve your daily routine.

6. Kettlebell Social Challenge

The Kettlebell Social Challenge transforms kettlebell training into an engaging and motivating social experience .

- **Key elements:**
    - Dedicated hashtags for each challenge (e.g. KettlebellWarrior2024).
    - Global and local leaderboards for various categories.
    - Fitness influencers as weekly mentors with live Q&A.
- **Gamification mechanics:**
    - Badges and achievements for various milestones.
    - Points system based on consistency, improvement and creativity.
    - Team challenges to promote mutual support.
- **User Generated Content:**
    - Contests for the most creative workout videos.
    - Transformation stories shared by the community .
    - Collaborations between users to create new challenges.

7. Kettlebell Mindfulness Fusion

Kettlebell Mindfulness Fusion is a holistic approach that combines the intensity of kettlebell training with mindfulness practices.

- **Program components :**
    - Pre and post workout guided meditation sessions.
    - Breathing exercises synchronized with kettlebell movements.
    - Visualization practices to improve performance.
- **Support Technology:**
    - App with biometric sensors to monitor stress levels.
    - Biodynamic audio feedback that adapts to your mental state.
    - Sleep analysis and tips to optimize recovery.
- **Benefits:**
    - Reduce stress and improve concentration.
    - Increase body awareness and prevent injuries.
    - Improving the balance between physical effort and mental well-being.

8. Kettlebell Family Fun

Kettlebell Family Fun is a program designed to engage the whole family in a fun and inclusive fitness journey.

- **Family Kit:**

- Kettlebell sets of various weights, including safe junior versions.
- Interactive mats with pressure sensors.
- Play accessories such as colored cones and inflatable obstacles.

- **Interactive App:**
    - Movement-based games that incorporate kettlebell exercises.
    - mode for family challenges.
    - Reward system that rewards the participation of all members.
- **Activity:**
    - "Kettlebell Treasure Hunt" - a fitness treasure hunt at home.
    - " Family Flow" - group routines that improve coordination.
    - "Strength Storytelling" - exercises integrated into interactive stories.
- **Benefits:**
    - Promoting an active lifestyle for all ages.
    - Strengthening family bonds through fitness.
    - Early education on the importance of physical exercise.

Each activity in this guide is designed to offer a fresh and engaging approach to kettlebell training, leveraging the latest fitness trends and technologies. Whether you're looking for an immersive experience, a personalized approach, or a way to get the whole family involved, these game-changing activities will help you transform your body and your workout routine.

5 Revolutionary Kettlebell Fitness Tips - Preview 2025

Are you ready to catapult your kettlebell training into the future? Here are 5 cutting-edge tips that promise to revolutionize your approach to fitness in 2025!

1. Kettlebell Neurofeedback Training

Tune your brain to your muscles!

In 2025, kettlebell training will not only be physical, but also neural. Get ready to empower your mind along with your body!

- How it works: Wear a sleek EEG headband while you work out. This cutting-edge technology monitors brain activity in real time.
- Benefits: Optimizes the mind-muscle connection, increasing movement efficiency and accelerating progress.
- Dedicated App: See in real time how your brain "lights up" during different exercises. Discover which movements activate the brain areas related to strength and coordination the most.
- Personalization: AI analyzes your neural patterns to suggest exercises that best suit your motor learning style.

Pro Tip: Start with short 10- minute sessions to get used to the neural feedback. Gradually increase the duration to maximize the mind-body benefits!

2. Anti-gravity Kettlebell

Defy gravity, push your limits!

Imagine being able to adjust gravity to your liking while exercising. In 2025, it won't be science fiction anymore!

- **Technology** : Advanced magnetic footplates that alter the perception of the weight of the kettlebell.
- **Mode** :
    - "Moon" (60% reduction in gravity)
    - "Mars" (40% reduction)

- "Jupiter" (20% increase)
- **Applications** :
    - Rehabilitation: Training with "lighter" weights without sacrificing movement.
    - Empowerment: Push yourself beyond your limits with increased gravity.
    - Intelligent Progression: AI adapts gravity in real time based on your performance, ensuring a constant challenge.

Pro Tip: Alternate sessions in different "gravities" for muscle and neural shock . Your body will never know what to expect!

3. Holographic Kettlebell with AI Coaching

Your personal 3D coach , always with you!

Forget 2D video tutorials. In 2025, your kettlebell coach will be an interactive hologram in your living room!

- **Immersive Experience** : High-definition holographic projections show correct exercise execution from every angle .
- **Voice Interaction** : Ask your AI coach to show a variation or slow down a specific move.
- **Real-time feedback** : AI analyzes your movements through environmental sensors, correcting your form instantly.
- **Advanced Personalization** : The AI coach adapts to your learning style, mood and daily energy level.

Pro Tip: Schedule "ghost sessions" where you and your holographic coach train side by side. Mimic their movements for perfect synchronization!

4. Eco-Adaptive Kettlebell

The kettlebell that grows with you, literally!

In 2025, your kettlebells will be alive and adapting to your needs. Welcome to the world of biotech fitness !

- **Revolutionary Material** : Organic polymers that change density and weight on command.
- **App Control** : Adjust the weight of your kettlebell from 2 to 40 kg with a simple swipe.
- **Eco Mode** : The kettlebell absorbs CO_2 from the air when you are not using it, helping to purify your home environment.
- **Biofeeback** : Built-in sensors measure your grip strength and adapt the surface texture for optimal grip.

Pro Tip: Use the "Progressive Overload" feature to automatically increase your weight by 1% each session. Steady growth, without thinking about it!

5. Social Augmented Reality Kettlebell

Train your body, connect your world!

By 2025, your kettlebell workout will be a global social experience, thanks to advanced augmented reality.

- **Ultra-lightweight AR glasses** : Put them on and transform your space into a shared virtual gym.
- **Global Group Workouts** : Join live sessions with people from all over the world, seeing them as if they were in your room.
- **Real-Time Challenges** : Compete in swing or snatch competitions with friends or strangers, viewing their avatars in AR.
- **Advanced Gamification** : Earn points, unlock achievements and conquer virtual locations with your performances.
- **3D Community Support** : Receive virtual high-fives and 3D encouragement from your global workout buddies.

themed workouts !

These tips are just a taste of what the future holds for kettlebell enthusiasts. In 2025, the line between physical and digital will blur, offering workout experiences we can only imagine today. Get ready to revolutionize not only your body, but your concept of fitness!

Glossary

1. **Kettlebell** : Ball-shaped exercise tool with a handle, used for dynamic and functional training. Excellent for increasing strength and cardiovascular resistance.

2. **Swing** : Basic kettlebell exercise in which you swing the kettlebell between your legs and then raise it to chest height , engaging the hamstrings, glutes, and core.

3. **Snatch** : Explosive lifting of the kettlebell from the ground above the head, used to improve strength and coordination.

4. **Clean** : Movement in which you lift the kettlebell from the floor to the rack position (on your chest), useful for preparing for other exercises such as the press.

5. **Press** : Exercise in which the kettlebell is raised above the head from the rack position, it mainly develops the shoulder and core muscles .

6. **Goblet Squat** : Squat performed while holding a kettlebell in front of the chest, strengthens the legs, glutes and core.

7. **Core** : Complex of muscles surrounding the torso and pelvis, essential for stability and balance.

8. **Metabolism** : The process by which the body converts food into energy. An active metabolism burns more calories, even at rest.

9. **Endurance : The body** 's ability to sustain physical exertion over time without tiring. Regular workouts increase endurance.

10. **Functional Strength** : The ability to perform everyday and athletic movements with greater efficiency and less risk of injury.

11. **HIIT (High-Intensity Interval Training) Training** : A series of short but intense exercises, alternating with periods of rest, ideal for burning fat quickly.

12. **Circuit Training** : Series of exercises performed one after the other without extended rests, designed to increase strength and endurance.

13. **Cardio** : Short for "cardiovascular training," focused on improving heart health and aerobic endurance .

14. **Fat burning** : Process by which the body uses stored fat as an energy source during physical activity.

15. **Posture** : Correct alignment of the body during movements and daily activities. Good posture reduces the risk of injury.
16. **Warm-up** : Light activity done before a workout to prepare the muscles and cardiovascular system for exercise.
17. **Cooldown** : A recovery activity performed at the end of a workout to help the body return to a resting state.
18. **Training Volume** : Total amount of work performed during a training session, usually measured in sets and repetitions.
19. **Set** : Group of repetitions of an exercise. For example, 3 sets of 10 repetitions.
20. **Repetitions** : The number of times an exercise is performed consecutively without rest.
21. **Range of motion** : The amount of joint movement during an exercise. The greater the range, the more muscles are involved.
22. **Progression : Gradual increase in** training intensity or load to stimulate physical adaptations.
23. **Overload** : Progressive overload used to stimulate increases in strength and muscle mass .
24. **Interval Training** : Training that alternates short periods of intense activity with moments of recovery, useful for improving aerobic and anaerobic capacity.
25. **Recovery** : The time it takes for muscles to repair and grow after a workout. It is essential to avoid overtraining.
26. **Overtraining** : A condition in which one exercises too much and without adequate rest, leading to chronic fatigue and reduced performance.
27. **Calories** : A unit of measurement for the energy contained in food. To lose weight, you need to consume more calories than you ingest.
28. **Balanced Diet** : A diet that provides all the essential nutrients in the right proportions to maintain optimal health and performance.
29. **Macronutrients** : Carbohydrates, proteins, and fats, the main components of the diet that provide energy.
30. **Protein** : Essential nutrient for muscle growth and repair, essential for kettlebell trainers.
31. **Complex carbohydrates** : Slow-release energy source, useful for supporting prolonged training and maintaining stable energy levels.

32. **Healthy Fats** : Unsaturated fats that provide energy and help the body function properly. They are found in foods such as avocado and olive oil.

33. **Calorie deficit** : Consuming fewer calories than needed to maintain your current weight, which is essential for losing fat.

34. **Cheat meal** : A planned meal where you eat foods that do not conform to your diet, useful for maintaining long-term motivation.

35. **Hydration** : Drinking enough water to maintain optimal body functions, especially during exercise.

36. **Overuse Injuries** : Injuries that occur when you exceed your workload or training frequency.

37. **Dynamic Stretching** : Active movements that lengthen muscles, ideal for preparing the body for an intense workout.

38. **Static stretching** : Muscle stretching technique while maintaining a fixed position, ideal after training to improve flexibility.

39. **Core Stability** : The ability of the core to stabilize the spine and pelvis during movement. Essential for improving performance and preventing injury.

40. **Squat** : Basic movement that mainly involves the muscles of the legs and glutes. Essential for functional strength.

41. **Deadlift** : An exercise that involves the entire body, especially the hamstrings , glutes, and back. Often used with kettlebells.

42. **Powerlifting** : Strength discipline that focuses on three exercises: squat, bench press and deadlift.

43. **PNF** (Proprioceptive Neuromuscular Facilitation) Stretching: Assisted stretching technique involving contraction and relaxation to increase flexibility.

44. **Muscle Isolation** : An exercise that involves a single muscle group, such as the biceps curl, as opposed to multi-joint functional exercises.

45. **Plyometric Exercise** : Explosive movements such as jumping or sprinting, ideal for improving power and speed.

46. **Interval Running** : Running technique that alternates sprints with periods of walking or slow running to improve speed and endurance.

47. **Body Fat Percentage** : The percentage of body fat relative to total body mass. It is a key indicator of physical health.

48. **Muscular endurance** : The ability of a muscle to sustain an activity for a prolonged period without tiring.

49. **EPOC** (Excess Post-Exercise Oxygen Consumption): Increased oxygen consumption after intense exercise , which helps burn calories even at rest.

50. **Functional training** : Exercises that simulate everyday or sports movements to improve functional capacity and prevent injuries.

Socrate

"It is a shame for a man to grow old without ever having seen the beauty and strength of which his body is capable."

Socrates, one of the fathers of Western philosophy, invites us to reflect on the hidden potential in our body, which we often ignore. Physical training is not just a matter of aesthetics or athletic performance, but a discovery of what we can achieve, both physically and mentally.

Cultivating physical strength, in fact, is an act of self-knowledge: through discipline and movement , we not only get closer to a better version of ourselves, but we realize the full expression of our human nature. Remaining inert means neglecting an essential part of our being.

* 9 7 9 8 3 0 3 9 9 0 1 6 6 *